IF I CAN JUST GET THROUGH THIS

IF I CAN JUST GET THROUGH THIS

A THERAPIST'S JOURNEY AND GUIDANCE THROUGH AUTISTIC SHUTDOWN AND ITS TRIGGERS

JESSICA C. KITCHENS

TABLE OF CONTENTS

Authors note

This book is written utilizing Neurodiversity-affirming language, including identity first language. While some background and reasoning may be discussed in this book based on certain topics, this author will not go into the extensive depth of these specific nuances but will gladly offer various other resources and books to point one in the right direction to increasing their neurodiversity-affirming knowledge at the end of this book.

INTRODUCTION

The need for this book came to me like a bolt of lightning one day on my way to work. It was January 2023, soon after the holidays, and I was cold and tired. This particular week was overbooked and overfilled in all areas. It was a Wednesday, which had become one of the busiest days of the week for my work. I had a song playing on repeat from Allman Brown called "Waiting for Something to Believe In." The part of the lyrics that kept sticking out to me was, "I'm tired, so tired of this… my soul's too heavy and I can't carry it." Somewhere along the route, a thought came as it often did: "If I can just get through this week." This was followed by the facetious thought that if there was ever a book about me, that would be the name of it.

Suddenly, my tiredness was replaced with an adrenaline rush. I had been working with a lot of clients recently on the topic of autistic shutdown, i.e., burnout and general triggers and recovery, and here I was struggling with my own. It only made sense to write about it from a therapist's perspective. And yes, that would be the name of the book. As it so happened, of the seven clients I had scheduled back to back that day, six were autistic, and four were struggling with issues related to autism shutdown. After each one, I wrote out notes to keep in mind the topics I wanted to highlight in this book.

That night, I wrote out an outline of the book, typed 8,000+ words, and got several chapters in. No, this is not typical for me. The next day, I wrote another 8,000 words only to be met with all my day's work getting accidentally deleted by a new program I attempted to use. What would have normally sent me straight to a meltdown was instead met with ten minutes of sitting in my room on the floor, having an internal dialogue about how pointless it would be to stop climbing a mountain if I fell and rolled back a bit. I came back out and started typing again, this time using the time-tested Google Doc. Those 8,000 words were replaced by 15,000 over the next couple of days. My husband and oldest daughter later told me they were quite surprised and proud of how I handled that setback. I suppose I was too, but something in me wasn't going to let me just stop. This needed to get out because it is a big struggle for many. One of the most common functional struggles for autistic adults, including myself.

When I was in graduate school for counseling, we were required to read *Man's Search for Meaning* by Viktor Frankl, a book I would highly recommend to anyone. One aspect of this book that I enjoyed was how the first half of the book was Frankl's story about his time in a Nazi concentration camp. It was especially important in order for you to understand where he was coming from in adapting his psychotherapeutic method, *Logotherapy,* discussed in the latter half of the book.

This book before you utilizes a similar principle; however, my story is interwoven within. An autistic's lived experience has always been fascinating to me. I find how past struggles and experiences might relate to present issues and current struggles to be especially imperative. I am exposing a great deal of vulnerability, and I hope you, as a reader, find some connection to it somewhere along the way. If anything, I hope if you struggle with shutdowns that, you are able to understand the thought processes behind them. Not everything will align with your lived experience, and that is okay. I hope you gain some insight even if you connect with my experience marginally.

CHAPTER ONE

HINDSIGHT OF THE AUTISTIC LENS

An autism diagnosis can often bring about an aspect of peace. For many late-diagnosed autistics, including myself, this is definitely the case. With this sense of relief, though, also comes the aspect of looking back on one's life through a whole new lens. This lens can bring about clarity to certain events and memories, but it can also bring about a variety of other complex and often difficult emotions. My therapy practice sees many clients at this crossroads in their autistic journey, and I now find myself at this same point.

As I look back at my life through the lens of an autism diagnosis, I am met with a mixture of heartache and perplexity as to how I made it through my formative years. The first half of my life was difficult, to say the least. My childhood was filled with more confusion than certainty, and my teenage years were turbulent in every way imaginable. Looking at my nine-year-old daughter who was diagnosed at the age of four, I definitely find myself envious of her free-spirited and uncaring nature. She is the unmasked version of me. I have learned more about myself in the past five years following her diagnosis than I learned in the 37 years prior. However, I also realize that the world now is not what it was then. I genuinely believe an earlier diagnosis for me would have introduced another veil of complexities into my life. Still, I would like to think it would have done so much for me to at least have known.

Looking back, I see a great many aspects of my childhood, teenage, and early adult years that I would have avoided had I been aware of my autism diagnosis. Some of this chapter may be difficult to read, so manage yourself accordingly, and please be aware of the trigger warnings present in the necessary sections. While many of these aspects are not necessarily related to shutdown, they are relevant to my journey and will be further discussed in the following chapters.

Looking Back

The thought that some individuals remember very little of their childhood has always confused me. I fall into another category of those who, for better or worse, remember practically everything. I did not have many talents as a child, but I do remember being an adept nap-taker. My grandmother, to whom we lived next door for a solid portion of my childhood, tells me she would often watch me walk into her house and fall asleep before my head hit the cushion.

Despite all that has changed since my childhood, I am still unable to get a good night's sleep most evenings, so I find naps to be one of the greatest gifts in creation—albeit a gift I can rarely accept due to the constant busyness of daily life. Even as a child, I deeply appreciated rest, both mental and physical. Realizing what I know now about the energy expenditure it takes to be autistic in a neurotypical world, I feel autistic individuals would benefit from understanding just how much rest we really need.

Through my childhood and teenage years, my energy expenditure ranged from that of a house cat dozing through the day to a squirrel frantically running and jumping from one place to another. I grew up living in the country, which I loved. My home was next to a heavily wooded area that I could explore with practically no limitations due to the free-range child-rearing attitude of the eighties.

As an eight-year-old, I would often ride my bike for several miles around the area lake. This is especially concerning due to our proximity to the Oklahoma State Penitentiary just a few miles down the road. The road itself was known for its frequent warning signs not to pick up hitchhikers, as escaped prisoners were not uncommon. Shockingly, I rarely knew fear and was never harmed, probably due in large part to my golden retriever, Precious, who accompanied me wherever I went. While these adventures were physically exhausting, I found them to be quite liberating. Despite the exhaustion, I was still unable to sleep much at night.

Not much changed when I entered school. I remember falling asleep on the bus both to and from school, then passing out on the couch as soon as I returned home. Despite my rather average academic performance, I struggled more than most to fit in and figure out what was going on around me. My internal confusion led to the constant need to mask, leading to even greater exhaustion.

I entered kindergarten at the age of four due to my birthday being in late August and the cut-off date for starting school being September 1st. One of my first memories of school was the teacher asking a question, to which most of the class responded by raising their hands. I had no clue why they were raising their hands, but I felt I should do the same. Elementary school was full of experiences such as this.

In contrast to my misunderstanding of conventional social cues, I had a strong justice principle from a very young age. I knew right from wrong and didn't understand why anyone would ever choose to do something that would get oneself into trouble. If I did get into trouble, it was typically for talking in class or some similar behavior that involved little insight or thinking. Many of these instances involved the breaking of unspoken rules or rules of which I had no awareness. Despite having no ill intentions, I was always filled with excessive shame and guilt, leaving me even more drained and exhausted than usual.

I transferred schools from a tiny school in third grade to a marginally bigger school in fourth. That transition was exceedingly difficult for me mentally, and it showed in my dropping grades. My new school proved to be an even more difficult adjustment as I also got my first taste of bullying from a handful of kids. My small stature made me a target, but looking back, I'm sure my awkwardness and hyperactivity played a role as well. Despite that, I did have friends and what I perceived to be an average social life.

I continued to be a target of cruelty from some peers through middle school and junior high. I noticed that it was particularly girls that exhibited these mean behaviors. I got along well with the boys and appreciated that they were easy to understand. On the other hand, the handful of girls who did not appear to like me were more difficult to understand. Sometimes, they would seem to be really sincere friends, only to turn on me without a discernible reason. The sheer mental exhaustion of it was starting to wear on me more, and I would actually mention it to my mom on occasion. She would try and sway my fears by telling me the typical things good moms say. Still, in the back of my mind, I knew I was different. I just did not understand how or why.

Over time, many of the girls who were mean to me ended up switching schools and were replaced by transfers, some of whom I knew before from my first elementary school. Ultimately, my highschool class was composed of about forty kids, a fourth of which was made up of girls. I found myself a small group of girls that I became especially close with. I have no doubt that if I had gone to a larger school, I would have struggled more to make friends. As it was, I got along with the majority of my class, boys and girls alike.

A big shift occurred in the middle of my junior year: I started feeling extreme exhaustion. I struggled to stay awake in classes, especially if they were before lunch. Teachers would try to wake me, and I would raise up only to put my head right back down and fall asleep. This was not a voluntary decision. I could not physically stay awake. It's a miracle I managed to get any school work done, albeit much of it was done last minute.

When I did manage to stay awake in class, I had a short fuse and was too exhausted to hide my displeasure. I even walked out of some classes as if there was no teacher there. I really do not know how I got away with that. In hindsight, it is clear that I was very dysregulated and attempting to avoid a public meltdown.

I felt very disconnected and out of it during this time. On one occasion, I remember walking down the hallway with a Walkman and headphones on. I felt like I was walking in slow motion while the rest of the world moved around me at this super fast pace. I know I looked like I was out of it because my guidance counselor saw me and called me out. She said something along the lines of if I needed to talk, to let her know. I just nodded.

All things considered, it's no surprise that I found no enjoyment in dating. I started seeing people around this time, mostly out of obligation and boredom, and it only added to my mental load. There was one particular relationship that I was unhappy in and tried to break off, only to be guilted into staying. My people-pleasing was in full effect at this time, and I remember feeling exhausted with even the idea of trying to break it off. So, I just tried to pull away in a slow fashion. This level of apathy and exhaustion led me to end the school year believing I was depressed, but I did not know what could be the cause. Looking back, I realize this was my first real episode of an autism shutdown.

Soon after that school year ended, my mother took me to a doctor, where I was diagnosed with extreme anemia. I was prescribed iron supplements and, within a few weeks, felt more like my normal self. I believe that shift had more to do with getting the rest I so desperately needed, in addition to finally leaving the relationship that I felt stuck in. I was happy to discover that he was cheating, allowing me to break it off with no remorse or guilt.

This being the summer prior to my senior year, I had to start making some decisions about my future. I knew one thing was for certain: I wanted to leave this place. While my parents were very hard-working individuals, unfortunately, neither were highly educated. This was something that both regretted but felt was never an option for them. I knew I wanted to go to college, but I had no guidance on how to go about it. The process of applying, coupled with the astronomical cost that my parents could in no way afford, felt like an insurmountable obstacle.

Rather than ask someone for help with my confusion surrounding college, I did what any reasonable person would do in this situation: I joined the Navy, signing up for the Delayed Entry Program at the beginning of my senior year. My brother was doing well in the Navy at that time, so it made sense. I knew it was an effective way to get college paid for. It also seemed ideal as I wasn't set on what degree to pursue, and this would allow me more time to decide. While I am not the best test taker on standardized tests in general, I scored very high on the pattern recognition part of the Armed Services Vocational Aptitude Battery (ASVAB). Because of that, I was going to train to become a CTR (Cryptologic Technician - Collection) after boot camp. I would have been doing coding of various types, apparently.

My decision to join the Navy had its pros and cons. On one hand, while all of my friends were busy filling out college applications and applying for scholarships, I was able to just coast along and did not even have to take the ACT. On the other hand, the repercussions of this decision would be evident in both my relationships and my mental health.

My senior year was an improvement from my junior year in many aspects, perhaps the most significant of which was my new relationship. I started dating a really great guy who, spoiler alert, would later become my husband. This school year was not without struggles, however. There were incidents where I would have what I called "assertive moments." My people-pleasing had left the building, and if someone was not being nice, I made sure to call them on it, sometimes in not-so-nice ways. Some of these incidents might be classified as aggressive meltdowns. One such meltdown occurred following an incident where a male classmate was speaking disparagingly about my friend, who was his ex, in front of me. This led to me yelling in his face and then walking away, followed by my first ever grand-mal/tonic-clonic seizure in the courtyard of our school. I had another seizure days later on my way home from school in my car. Luckily, I had an aura and knew something was not right, so I pulled over. I do not remember how I got home, but I know it involved friends. This was long before the days of cell phones, so I couldn't have even called for help. Following these seizures, my mom took me for an EEG in hopes of finding their cause. During this test, I was meant to fall asleep. However, I was unable to despite staying up all the previous night. Thus, the test yielded no results. I did not disclose any information about my seizures to my recruiter as I believed that they were simply flukes.

As the end of my highschool career and the beginning of my military career neared, my anxiety rose. My paternal grandmother tried to sway me from going to boot camp by offering to help me get a car and get into college. My shame meter would not allow me to accept the offer. For one, I did not want to put that on her, and two, I did not want to go back on my word to my recruiter. I know, silly.

And so I graduated at 17. I enjoyed my last summer reluctantly before I had to leave in September, a month after turning eighteen. I grew more ambivalent about having to go, and while I knew I had to, I really did not want to leave Steven, my boyfriend. I continued to work out, and as usual, I took many naps. Inevitably, my time ran out, and I had to leave. I would come to regret my choice to not ask questions about my options and, perhaps even more so, to not have prepared a backup plan.

THE NAVY AND A HIDDEN DIAGNOSIS

When the time came for me to leave, I was consumed with both fear and excitement, but mostly fear. I realize now that the overwhelming fear was actually anxiety, and it has never really left me since.

Upon my arrival in Chicago in the middle of the night, I was thrown into the culture shock of non-civilian living. I immediately went through the motions of being processed, which included getting a haircut and collecting my items. There were many other details I do not remember from this because I have dissociated and blocked them out. My lack of memory is also due in part to the fact that I was severely sleep-deprived.

As if the stress of exhaustion and lack of familiarity wasn't enough, I had also started my period the night before my plane ride. Throughout the hours I was being processed, I had no access to feminine hygiene products or even a restroom. The extreme discomfort further exacerbated my dysregulation.

On two occasions, I asked my superiors for hygiene products and the opportunity to go to the restroom. "You will soon get that opportunity," I was told both times. That opportunity didn't come until hours later. I was standing in line with other women, drowning in feelings of desperation and a lack of control. I mustered up what little courage I could to speak out at the nearest Master Chief Petty Officer: "I really need to go to the restroom to take care of my period, Petty Officer Sir!" He must have sensed my distress because he went into a room and returned with a hygiene product.

Once inside the bathroom stall, I was able to inspect the damage. It was bad. Hours of no control over my environment and extreme stress had taken their toll on my body, and the inside of my military PT (Physical Training) sweats were evidence of that. While the feeling of panic consumed me, a small part of me was appreciating the inner mesh layers that had prevented the outside from showing the damage the inside had taken.

I coached myself into holding it together. I couldn't let anyone know something was off. The amount of masking required during this was excessive, and my capability to hold it together despite the dysregulation I felt and the sleep-deprived sensory hell I was in is really impressive in hindsight; however, it is also exceedingly sad at the same time. I still get very emotional when I think back on this time.

It was several more hours before we were allowed into our barracks, and I once again had to gather the courage to approach a room full of mostly male petty officers and request permission to change clothes. Their prying eyes told me they were not pleased with whatever was going on. I requested to speak to a female petty officer to explain. It was later announced to our whole barracks that, as women, we needed to trust the male petty officers enough to make the same requests as we would from a female petty officer. I knew that announcement was made due to my actions, and I did not care, honestly. I was simply happy to be back with clean items.

By the time we were unpacked, showered, and getting ready for bed, it had been 19 hours since my arrival and my first opportunity to sleep. It had been nearly two days since I had last slept. While many were able to drop their head and sleep briefly on a desk while waiting through processing, I was not one of the lucky ones who could fall asleep easily enough to do so. This was the same brain that gave me insomnia most nights and did not allow me to fall asleep for my EEG.

In all of my preparation for boot camp life, nothing had prepared me or my brain for this. I remember finally being able to fall asleep, so exhausted due to all that had transpired that I didn't have the energy to worry.

What happened next is still somewhat of a mystery to me. I had flashes of an ambulance ride and bits of memory of being in a hospital. Nothing tangible to relate to what was happening to me. It was later conveyed to me in the hospital that I had a seizure in my sleep. Apparently, it was a pretty violent one, as I was told by others in my barracks that I had kicked a Petty Officer as she pulled me out from under the bed.

While in the hospital, I was prescribed Dilantin, an anti-epileptic medication that inhibited my short-term memory. I hated it and the awful brain fog it caused. The amount they had me on was exceedingly high, and they never tried anything else. Perhaps it was the standard they used in the military, but I am aware now that there are a lot of different medications for seizures.

I vaguely remember making my way back to my barracks in a white van in the dark. I don't know what time it was or how much time had passed. My splotchy memory also includes trying to talk to a couple of young recruits who were on watch. I was trying to tell them that I needed to get back into my barracks, but I had no idea where in the building my division was located. I know my words were slurred from the Dilantin, and I am sure I appeared very under the influence. Somehow, they located where I was supposed to be, and I got back in bed.

The next few days were a blur. My brain felt fried. Functioning at my best was maybe 40% of what I was generally capable of, and this limited me on many levels. My medication made me very sleepy, which combined with the limited time I had to sleep, resulted in more seizures. It's ironic that my seizure medication only made things worse. In just over a week's time, I had approximately seven seizures. One was even on a staircase. My last memory included me going up the stairs holding one of the flags (why I was picked for this honor, I do not know). I was later told that I had fallen all the way down to the bottom. The bruises covering my body were evidence that it was not a light fall. Although I had a gut feeling before this particular seizure occurred, I had hoped I could make it to the barracks before it happened. Yet again, I let fear win and fell into my pattern of masking instead of asking for help.

Shortly after my fall down the stairs, reality came crashing down as well: I was informed that seizure disorders are not allowed in the military and therefore, I would be discharged. Upon hearing this, I felt numb. I don't think I was able to fully comprehend what that meant at the time due in part to the Dilantin.

I was told to pack my things and was transferred to a different barracks called separations, where those who were being discharged resided. Many were there because of major injuries sustained in PT, while others were there due to failure to comply or mental issues.

Separation from the military appeared to be a very lengthy process. The simpler the issue was, the quicker the discharge; however, even those could take weeks, and there were many individuals who had been stuck there for months. Months away from home with limited contact with their loved ones. Perhaps worse than being stuck in limbo for an excessive period of time was simply having no idea just how long it would be. The only indication that home was right around the corner was having your name written on the board.

Time crawled due to my confusion, boredom, and numbness from the medication. I had not heard from my family since I spoke to my mother briefly after first arriving. They were completely oblivious to everything that had transpired up to this point, as the Navy didn't seem to think my multiple hospital visits were worthy of a call home. After hours of being in separations, though, I was finally allotted the privilege.

The minute the phone hit my hand and I heard my mother's voice, the mask I had tried so hard to uphold crumbled. I had only a few minutes to relay everything that had happened, and it all came out in a jumbled, sobbing mess as I had a full-fledged meltdown. I was scared and confused and wanted nothing more than to be anywhere but where I was. My medication limited my explanation of things, and my poor mom was left terrified when I had to hang up. Having been hit with all the emotions I had suppressed since my arrival, I was unable to calm down. I had another seizure resulting in another ambulance trip I don't remember.

A week passed with no answers. During that time, I was restricted from leaving the barracks due to seizure precautions. I mostly stayed in bed and read. I tried to limit my stress and sleep when I could. This limited my seizure activity to only one during my sleep.

One day, while reading on my cot, a couple of outside young recruits approached me. I was told to dress up in what I call the "Smurf" uniform: a light blue button-up shirt tucked into dark blue pants. I was not told why, just to do it. I followed these men out of the building to a much further away office building. I was then told to wait outside of a Master Chief Petty Officer's office with several other recruits. Confusion and fear twisted into a knot in my stomach. Several anxiety-laden minutes later, the Master Chief came out and asked which one of us was Jones. That was me (my maiden name). He led me into his office and then waited for the phone to ring. He answered, speaking briefly to the individual on the other end, and then directed me to sit in his desk chair before handing me the phone. He then left his own office. That was really odd to me, and I did not know what to expect on the other end of that phone. The voice I heard was someone I least expected: my cousin Monty.

My cousin was highly ranked as an officer. I do not remember what he was at that time, but he retired as a Captain in 2022. Once I realized it was family on the other end, my mask again fell, and my emotions got the best of me. I began sobbing once again. He asked me questions, and I tried to answer them the best I could. I remember telling him I just wanted to go home. The conversation was brief, but it was less rushed than the one with my mother. Apparently, it was she who called him to try and get some answers. It was all she knew to do. He was able to speak to others on my behalf about the situation and was then able to relay to my mom more information that she otherwise would not have gotten from me. But more importantly, that call got my name on the board the next day, which meant I was going home in 2-3 days. The sense of relief I felt cannot be explained. I owe my cousin so much. I still do not know how to thank him.

HEADING HOME TO DESPAIR

Despite losing my spending and ID cards during one of my ER visits, I was able to recover the money that remained. It was not easy, though, and the military personnel who assisted me did not hide their displeasure with me for losing them in the first place. I thought it was ridiculous that they blamed me for losing something while I was seizing and unconscious, but I kept my thoughts to myself. The lack of grace at times was more than a little upsetting, but ableism in the military is really not that surprising.

With my tickets in hand, I was dropped at the O'Hare International Airport. While I was accompanied by several other individuals who were also blessed to be going home, I was not provided an official guide to help me in my fairly drugged state. Once inside, I went to a McDonald's and got the biggest meal I could. My diet in boot camp and separations was sparse, consisting mostly of rice, fruit, and occasionally fish. Sinking my teeth into a double-quarter pounder after weeks of bland food was transformational. If freedom had a taste, that is what it would taste like.

While roaming the airport in search of my terminal, I bought a Stephen King book from the bookstore to read on the plane. In spite of my drugged and overwhelmed state, I managed to find my gate. I boarded the plane and fell asleep before we had even taken off. So much for that book.

Upon landing in Oklahoma City, I was greeted by my paternal grandparents. Words can't describe how relieved I felt to see familiar faces. They took me to Red Lobster, where I was once again reminded of what I had been missing. I don't recall much of the conversation from dinner or the hours-long ride that followed, but I do remember that they were very supportive of me. Hearing how much they loved and missed me lifted a weight off of my shoulders.

After they dropped me off, I called Steven and told him I was home. He arrived at my house in the exact 15 minutes it took to get there. When we hugged, I felt safe for the first time in weeks.

The next morning, my plan was to sleep as long as I could. I awoke at 11:00 a.m., which compared to the 4:00 a.m. wake-up I was accustomed to, was heaven. It's crazy how something that had been routine for years felt so foreign after only a few weeks. Gone were the barracks and unsympathetic petty officers. There I lay in my childhood bedroom, enveloped in the quiet of an empty home. A thought pierced through the silence: "What now?" Never had I imagined I would be back home so soon and under such circumstances. I never considered a backup plan; I was left directionless. After spending a few days catching up with Steven and friends, my mom told me I should start looking for a job.

I agreed to get a job. However, there proved to be an unforeseen obstacle standing in my way: an extreme level of anxiety. While I had experienced anxiety my entire life, it was a functional anxiety that directed me to get things done and would dissipate after the task was finished. This was constant, though. I so desperately wanted to put the nightmare that was my time in the Navy behind me, but the trauma of my experience continued to haunt me. I was not only experiencing unprecedented levels of anxiety but also suffering from the brain fog from my Dilantin.

These struggles hindered my job search. I would apply for jobs, but it was difficult to perform the tasks necessary to keep working. Such was the case when I was hired to be a server, contingent on my ability to memorize the menu. After several days of trying my best to accomplish this, I had made very little progress. I knew my efforts were futile and gave up. Overwhelmed both by my inability to perform basic tasks and the stress of finding direction, I fell into a depression.

I fell deeper into my depression as the feeling of failure crept in. All the plans I had made to leave my hometown, go to college, and make a better life for myself had come crashing down, and I had no idea how to go about picking up the pieces. I tried to distract myself by spending time with Steven and my friends, but over time, I started to feel like I was pulling them down with me.

I felt myself struggling to function under the crushing weight of all my failures. One particular evening, my mom was griping me out in the kitchen about not getting a job. I just sat there, despondent and unmoving. I stared at the microwave with a face of stone and did not respond. I didn't tell her that I already felt like a failure. I didn't tell her that hearing what I needed to do wasn't helping. I didn't tell her that there was nothing she could say that was worse than I had already thought about myself. I simply made the silent decision to leave that night. I loaded up my car and left through my window after everyone had fallen asleep. My married friend, Charlette, allowed me to stay with her, and I immediately felt like a burden to her and her husband as well. I knew I needed to make a change.

It was around this time that I ran into my friend, Eddie, at Walmart. At one point, our conversation turned to my situation with leaving the Navy due to my seizures and how I wasn't sure what to do next. As luck would have it, he had a Vocational Rehabilitation

Grant for his asthma that helped pay for his college, and he said I might apply for it as well. He gave me the name of his Vocational Rehab counselor, Arthur McMullen, and I finally felt a flicker of hope.

One phone call with McMullen later, I was sitting in his office feeling scared but optimistic. He looked at my DD214 military discharge papers and told me that because my seizures caused me to have to come home after trying to be out on my own, I could now use my own income to get approved versus my parents'. This was good news since my parents' income was too high to get approved, and it also meant that I was eligible for the PELL grant. He got the ball rolling quickly, and I was able to apply to the local college and start classes in January. I cannot express how grateful I was for his help.

When applying for college, I had to choose a major for my paperwork. I had no clue what I wanted to do. I had always liked the idea of being a forensic detective or a profiler, so I chose criminal justice. It didn't really matter what major I chose initially since all of my first semester classes were just the basics. Though things were looking up with my classes starting, my depression persisted.

I had thought to myself that if I could just do something worthwhile, be it getting a job or pursuing a degree, all of the negative feelings bogging me down would disappear. However, starting college made me realize this was not the case. It was, if anything, a small bandage on a gaping wound. I was still struggling mentally with my cognitive loss from my medicine. Classes were hard. Focusing was impossible. I felt even more burdensome.

All of these factors led me to the decision to break up with Steven for his benefit. As I explained to him how I felt like a burden and did not want to trouble him, I had hoped he would reassure me that things would be okay. That is not how the conversation played out, though. He told me that he wasn't in a good place either. Guilt consumed me as I felt that I was the cause. This reinforced to me that I was making the right decision.

Things started to go downhill following Steven and I's breakup. I started to make decisions that were very out of character for me. For one, my friend's house that I was staying at had alcohol available, and I did not stay away from it despite the fact that I wasn't even fond of the stuff. On top of that, I started seeing someone new, "Ethan," shortly after our split. Steven and I had broken up a few times in the past, and all of those times, he had been the one to quickly rebound. This was the first time that it was the other way around.

Unaware of my new relationship, Steven reached out to me and told me that he wasn't doing well. He expressed that he regretted our breakup and was taking part in self-destructive behaviors as a result. Guilt set in, and I felt responsible for his actions. Due to my justice principle, I felt that it was my job to fix the situation. Despite knowing that I was in an unhealthy place, I chose to get back together with him and break it off with Ethan. At least, that was the plan. My people-pleasing tendencies allowed me to be guilted into staying in that relationship as well.

Mistake after mistake, guilt and shame accumulated and overwhelmed me. These emotions are the most difficult ones to encounter, and for good reason: they are meant to motivate an individual to stop certain behaviors. They are like a pressing weight that cripples the mind, hence why I call them the heaviest of emotions. No person is strong enough to resist their weight for long. The pain can be numbed by substances or distractions but not avoided– only delayed. Guilt and shame rise like a raging river, and eventually, the dam holding them back breaks. Then, it's sink or swim.

The Perfect Storm

(Trigger warning: Mention of suicidal thoughts and attempts are discussed in this chapter. Feel free to continue to the next chapter if you need to manage yourself.)

When Steven was eight, he had a bike accident that resulted in a bad bruise on his hip. He didn't think much of it and carried on with typical eight-year-old activities, including swimming in the lake. A short time later, he became extremely ill with a high fever that wouldn't go away. The doctors discovered that his bruise had become infected after exposure to bacteria in the lake. The infection was deep in his bone; it could not be treated with a simple round of antibiotics; rather, it required a major surgery wherein they drilled down into his bone and left the wound open to heal.

Looking back on my early adult years, I realize that I was like a bruise, open to infection. I was made vulnerable by my circumstances, including extreme exhaustion, medical crises, and the feeling of failure, as all of my plans fell through. These traumas made way for feelings of shame and guilt to creep in, creating a perfect storm that made me fall deep into depression. As it was for Steven's case, the solution to my situation would not be simple or painless.

Things got worse before they got better. I had entered the territory of seeing two men at the same time, one of whom I loved and felt I needed to save and the other whom I had no desire to be with but did not know how to break things off. I tried on multiple occasions to firmly end things with Ethan, but he made it difficult. One of my attempts to break up with Ethan ended in him fabricating a health crisis to garner sympathy from me and guilt me into staying. I felt like a rope being pulled apart at the seams, always on the verge of snapping.

I felt that I had no control over my own life, and I didn't know how to take back the reins. All of my relationships were plagued with pain and unmet expectations. Part of me started to believe that I was the common denominator in everyone's suffering. That lie took root and grew until I considered it a fact. I wanted to save everyone, and I thought that the only way to do that was to take myself out of the equation. I started to plan to do just that.

The morning of my plan, I woke up despondent. Charlette and I were alone at the time in her house. To my surprise, Steven showed up early that morning. This struck me as odd because it was a school day, and he was still a senior. Adding to my concern was his upset demeanor. Once we were alone, he confronted me about Ethan, as he had learned the truth from a friend. Because of my decision to take my life that day, I am ashamed to say that I denied the accusations. As much as I hated to lie, I rationalized doing so by telling myself that soon I would right the situation by removing myself from it.

After he left, I went to the store and purchased some CDs. I specifically sought songs that were not healthy for my mindset. I then drove to my parent's home. As I went through the motions of carrying out my plan, I didn't think the gravity of the situation had hit me. I felt nothing. It was like I was checking off an ordinary to-do list. Go to my room and shut the door. Check. Turn on the music and crank the volume. Check. Down a full bottle of OTC painkillers and all of my remaining Dilantin. Check. Go to bed early. Check.

Closing my eyes, I thought that was it. I had no intention of ever waking up. I sank into unconsciousness, at peace with dying.

I awoke hours later to my mother bringing me the phone. I was disoriented and didn't even have time to process the failure of my plan before Steven was in my ear, yelling and cursing me out. News had spread that I was seeing someone else, and it was impossible to deny it at that point. I listened and did not argue. My brain was foggy and tired from the drugs, and I simply wanted the conversation to be over like everything else. "I am letting you go now," I told him. I meant it as an apologetic goodbye, but he did not take it that way. "No, I'm letting you go!" He shot back before hanging up the phone. I felt even more sure about my decision after this.

I grew more and more impatient as the hours ticked by. I had hoped that things would move a lot quicker than this. Despite the fact that I was nowhere near sober enough to be behind the wheel,

I decided to drive to Charlette's house. I knew that her husband had a gun there. She and her husband were fast asleep, so I was able to locate the gun without their noticing.

Pistol in hand, I stepped outside onto the front porch. Standing alone in the cool night air, I had every intention to end it all. With the pull of a finger, it would be over in an instant. Thoughts of indecision clouded my mind, though. I thought about Charlette and her husband who would discover my body. I also thought about my mother, who I had promised upon my departure that I would be back in the morning to watch my sister. With these things in mind, I froze.

Those few moments of hesitation were interrupted by Ethan pulling up. The events that transpired after his arrival are a blur. I sat outside on the porch for a while until I was hit with the urge to throw up. I slept on the bathroom floor that night. I don't know what happened to the gun, but I am sure that Ethan wisely did something with it.

I awoke the next day feeling more clear-headed but unbelievably sick. Rather than spend the day recovering, I forced myself to attend my college computer applications class that night after watching my younger sister during the day. It was a punishment, I thought to myself, for putting myself into this position. I had made myself sick so I would reap the consequences. At some point during the class, I was hit with another round of nausea, so I left class to head to the restroom. However, what happened after I left the room, including whether or not I even made it to the restroom, remains a mystery to me as I blacked out.

When I opened my eyes, I was in the ER. I had a seizure despite all of the Dilantin in my system, resulting in the college calling an ambulance. Labs showed that I had a terrible kidney infection and a dangerous amount of Dilantin in my system, so the doctors wanted to admit me. I was aware of both of these issues prior to my hospital visit. I knew I had an infection a week prior, but as I had no insurance and did not want to burden my parents, I numbed the pain with AZO. This led to the infection spreading to my kidneys. I tried to refuse admittance as I was an adult, but my dad sternly told me, "You're staying!"

It was the infection that had caused my seizure. Had I not forced myself to go to school, it would have occurred at home, and my parents would not have called an ambulance. The kidney infection, coupled with the Dilantin slowly poisoning my body, would have eventually killed me.

While in the hospital, no social worker came to speak to me. No suicide assessment was ever given. Whether they were truly or willfully ignorant of my intentions, I'll never know for sure. Their lack of due diligence, though, left me at risk as I still intended to rectify my failure. I still had no hope. Nothing had changed. If anything, I felt worse and even more burdensome than before.

Pushing Through

(Trigger warning: The mention of pregnancy loss is discussed in this chapter. Feel free to continue to the next chapter if you need to manage yourself.)

Upon being discharged from the hospital, I was told by doctors that I could not drive due to my risk of seizures. As a result, I had to rely on friends and family to get around. This meant that I was constantly with someone. I was still in a very vulnerable state, and I'm not sure if anyone knew the truth behind my hospitalization. If they did, no one ever addressed the elephant in the room except for my friend Jaime. She had moved over an hour away a few years prior, but she still called to check in on me. She asked me outright if I had tried to take my life. Filled with shame, I lied. I hate that I let the stigmatization around suicide prevent me from reaching out for help, but her even asking the question did snap me awake a bit.

Shortly after being discharged, my friend Charlette picked me up to go to her house. They had heard through the grapevine that Steven was once again taking part in self-destructive behaviors. It broke my heart to hear that he was in such a dark place, but I realized that in spite of my sadness and guilt, there was nothing I could do to fix his situation. I had previously made plans with him to come drop off my things at Charlette's house. I knew that I was not ready to face him, so I made sure to be out of the house when he came by.

When I later returned, I discovered that Steven had not returned all of my things. There were a few important items missing, one of which was a rare teddy bear that my grandma had given to me. My desire to reclaim these sentimental items outweighed my desire to avoid seeing Steven, so I convinced Charlette to drive me to his house. She was hesitant to do so, given the rumors she had heard, but she ultimately agreed.

When I arrived, I found that Steven was also staying with friends. I asked to speak with him, so he came outside. His cold demeanor and defensive words were not surprising to me.

Not in the mood to argue, I calmly asked him for the rest of my stuff. He told me he had burned them. I felt gut-punched. I ached to think of all the treasured things I would never see again, but a part of me felt that he was justified in his actions. "I guess I deserved that," I thought whilst staring at the ground.

I listened silently as he tore into me, at times offering an apology for what I could. All of the hurt from the last couple of months came tumbling out in a whirlwind of harsh words. Charlette tried to get me to leave, but I forced myself to hear what he had to say in hopes that it would bring him closure. It was the least I could do.

Eventually, the angry words dwindled. Steven seemed to have gotten it all out of his system, sounding more like his usual self as the conversation progressed. Charlette had grown tired of waiting and told me that she wanted to go home. To my surprise, Steven offered to take me home in her stead. She did not look comfortable leaving me there, but I told her that I would be fine. I felt hopeful that this was a sign that Steven did not hate me anymore. With concern in her eyes, Charlette left.

Steven and I continued to talk. I answered his questions as honestly as I could, although I was unable to express the depths of my struggle with depression. With the benefit of hindsight, I know now that my inability to put this into words stemmed from my struggles with pragmatics and aphasia from the seizures. At the time, though, I think it was easier for him to see my behaviors without understanding the reasons behind them.

We had been talking for a while when Charlette returned, this time with another friend of mine, Amber. They jumped out of the car and immediately started yelling at me. Fearing that Steven was a bad influence, they were determined to get me away from him. They demanded that I leave with them for my own well-being. I yelled back at them that I did not want to leave. I felt perfectly safe with Steven, and I didn't need their interference. However, they were undeterred. They were determined to "rescue" me by any means necessary. Amber grabbed me by my sweatshirt and started to pull me in the direction of the car. I resisted. This game of tug-of-war ended with her pulling off my sweatshirt, leaving me dazed in my bra and jeans.

The demand from others, it seemed, was neverending. For months, my life had been spiraling out of control, leaving me feeling powerless and drained. What I wanted seemed to always be just out of sight, obscured by the demands of others. There I stood, wanting nothing more than to stay with Steven and continue to patch things up, but once again, it felt like my feelings were trumped by what others wanted me to do. With these thoughts clouding my mind, I snapped.

Blinded by both my tears and rage, I told them I was done and turned to leave. In the distance, I could see my destination: the highway. I wanted the demand from others to stop. Permanently. I trudged towards the road, half-naked and in complete meltdown, with every intention to walk out into traffic.

Unaware of my plan, Steven diffused the situation with Charlette and Amber and got them to leave. He caught up to me before I ever made it to the road and took me inside the house. I'm not sure how long it took for him to calm me down, but he eventually did. Once I felt more regulated, he drove me home.

The drive from Steven's house to mine was usually about fifteen minutes. It was the dead of night, and we were cruising on the dirt back roads. At some point during the drive, I noticed that there were headlights following us. The closer we got to my house, the closer the lights got. Steven started to drive faster in order to lose them, but to no avail. My fear quickly turned to anger as I realized that this was likely connected to the events that had previously unfolded.

When we pulled up to my home, I told Steven to park around the back. I hopped out of his car and stormed around to the front of the house, where the car that had been following us parked. Inside was Ethan and Charlotte's husband. They had heard from Amber and Charlotte about Steven driving me home and followed us, supposedly out of concern. All of the anger that I had swallowed from earlier increased tenfold. I tore into them, telling them that they were stupid for following me and that they needed to leave immediately.

The days following this incident were difficult. My friends were mad at me. I was mad at myself for letting things get to this point.

This led to me doing something that I should have done months prior: I prayed and submitted the whole situation to God. I stopped trying to fix everything and realized that I needed to relinquish my desire to control things that I couldn't. I had no idea where to go moving forward, but I told God that I was open to whatever plan he had laid out for me. This decision filled me with a peace and clarity of mind that I had previously been missing. I also stopped taking Dilantin for good, which I believe improved my mental state.

With this renewed clarity, I saw how my mind had been fooled both by my depression and by the manipulations of other people. I started to work on improving all areas of my life, including myself and my relationships. During this time, Steven was able to work past his own problems and forgive me, and we were once again trying to make things work as a couple. That summer, we found out we were expecting.

Initially very frightened by this revelation, we quickly became excited. Although we were young, unmarried, and naive, pregnancy woke us up very quickly, and we started to plan our future together. Steven had gotten accepted to a university a couple hours away, where he received a full-ride scholarship. I transferred there, too. We decided to get married in August, the same month that classes started. We kept our plans and pregnancy hidden briefly before breaking the news to our parents. Thankfully, they handled it well.

A short time after telling our parents, I woke up one morning bleeding heavily. Following a fainting spell, my mom took me to the ER. After performing an ultrasound, they told me that they were unable to locate anything and that I had miscarried. Devastation does not even begin to describe how I felt. Despite the support I had from Steven and family, the grief and guilt hurt terribly. Everywhere I looked was a reminder of what I had lost. I felt that this was a punishment for my bad decisions. I thought that I deserved this pain.

In spite of our difficult loss, Steven and I wanted to continue with our plans to get married. We had limited time before school started, so things were pretty rushed. We got married on August 14th, and we moved into married student housing and started classes just over a week later. On August 23rd, I turned nineteen. Only a year prior, I had joined the Navy around this time. The year I became an adult, I was faced with the darkest and most difficult year of my life.

My nineteenth year was not without difficulties, but I at least felt direction and hope once again. After transferring schools, I took an Interviewing Techniques course that I thought was about interviewing criminals, however, it turned out to be a counseling class detailing the topic of motivational interviewing. It was in that class that I realized that I wanted to pursue becoming a therapist, and I changed my major soon after.

We later discovered that we were expecting again, but this time with twins. We lost one around thirteen weeks. Devastated once again, I pushed through knowing I still had one growing. Gage was born in September just after I turned twenty.

The 20+ years that followed were filled with a whirlwind of events. Steven and I both graduated with our bachelor's degrees in 2003. I graduated with a degree in Human Services Counseling, and Steven graduated with a degree in Chemistry. We moved to Northwest Arkansas the August following graduation for Steven's graduate program at the University of Arkansas.

Our second child, Kieran, was born the December after we moved to Arkansas. I started graduate school for counseling in 2005. Our third child, Ryker, was born in the midst of all that in September of 2006. My youngest two children, Heston and Ridlee, were born at home several years later in 2011 and 2014. A lot happened in those years that have brought me to where I am now.

CHAPTER TWO

WHAT IS AUTISTIC SHUTDOWN?

ll individuals deal with stress, regardless of whether you are an autistic or an allistic (non-autistic) individual. Everyone has a threshold as to how much stress they can endure before it begins to affect one's basic ability to function. This threshold can change day by day depending on a number of different variables. Shutdowns, often interchangeable with the term burnout, are a neurological response in the form of an involuntary internal pause button. Some resources claim that burnout is simply a long-term manifestation of a shutdown. I would argue that they are the same in terms of biological triggers and symptoms, as well as prevention and treatments.

The semantics of this particular subject are not crucial to the larger point that I am trying to get across. Therefore, when I use them in the context of this book, I consider the two to be synonymous.

A shutdown typically occurs as a method for the brain to protect itself. This may look like an acute shutdown over a trigger that occurs unexpectedly, like a sensory or cognitive overload. On the other hand, the shutdown may manifest as a gradual slowing of mental processes over time when consistent demands are placed on one for far too long. I have always considered shutdowns to be like a computer slowing or stopping auxiliary processes in order to prioritize basic functions.

If you research autistic shutdown or burnout, you will see a lot of information on the subject, but mostly in regard to children who are affected and what to do as a parent or caregiver. While this is important, there is not nearly enough information out there in terms of struggling through this as an adult. In both adults and children, a shutdown is generally discussed in brief detail or in short blogs and does not go into nearly enough detail. There are some autistic advocates who offer training on the subject, but I have not had the opportunity to partake in those at the time of writing.

What is particularly confusing about this is the fact that autistic shutdowns are one of the most significant and most common struggles for autistic adults to contend with. Without proper support and positive coping mechanisms, shutdowns inevitably lead to decreased overall functioning, increased likelihood of meltdowns, and increased likelihood of other mental health difficulties. While an allistic adult can reach a point where they are led to a similar response of shutdown, the brain of an autistic adult is far more vulnerable due to the overwhelming nature of daily life in the modern world. This essentially means that autistic adults reach the threshold of shutdown far quicker than neurotypical adults.

These specific environments are often the reason that some people struggle more as adults than kids or teenagers. One must also consider that our environment is always changing, now more so than ever. In the past two decades, the increase in technology, infrastructure, businesses, and population has added to the increasingly complicated and overstimulating environments that an autistic brain may struggle with. This is one reason why there are more adults being diagnosed with autism later in life than ever before; that and the fact that we are finally becoming more knowledgeable about what autism really is and how vast that spectrum can be.

SYMPTOMS: WHAT DOES AN AUTISTIC SHUTDOWN LOOK LIKE IN ADULTS?

Shutdown often creeps in gradually. Autistics don't usually wake up one day and find themselves in total shutdown. The beginning signs are often ignored. One day, you may find yourself more exhausted than usual, even though you thought you got decent sleep. And because of this, your energy takes a hit. Or maybe you are finding yourself more frustrated or irritable being around people. Sometimes, the simple notion of being around others seems daunting. On these days, I find myself thinking, "I don't want to people today." Maybe your patience is becoming non-existent, even with basic tasks.

Other symptoms might include being more sensitive to sensory overload, difficulty with simple tasks, or finding certain words that are much more labor-intensive than they should be. Regulating one's emotions often becomes more arduous during a shutdown.

Some individuals also describe symptoms of dissociation during a shutdown, which I have also experienced personally. Many of these symptoms are a result of autistic shutdown's effect on the prefrontal cortex. As far as shutdown triggers go, both acute and chronic stress can impair executive functioning, which resides in the prefrontal cortex (Arnsten, 2009).

It's also notable that autistic individuals struggle more with executive dysfunction than neurotypical individuals. So, it is no wonder that autistic regression often occurs during times of shutdown or why we may get there sooner. If both acute and chronic stress affects executive functioning, an autistic individual is going to struggle more with daily tasks, such as basic communication, planning, and paying attention. In addition, shutdown may lead to lapses in reasoning, working memory, cognitive flexibility, and impulse control, as well as an increase in rigid thinking (Hughes et al., 1994). When working memory is affected, cognitive overload — when too much information is presented at once, inhibiting the ability to process it all— is more likely to occur.

When autistics try to simply push through these early symptoms of shutdown, their executive functions are increasingly negatively affected as time goes on. Many autistics have comorbid physical disabilities as well. Symptoms of these are most likely to increase during shutdowns. This is one reason why autism is described as a dynamic disability. This basically means that an autistic individual's symptoms, abilities, and support needs can change from day to day. The varying ability to function as an autistic adult leads many within the autistic community to feel that autism should not be described using functioning labels.

The Problem with Functioning Labels

According to the newest addition of the Diagnostic and Statistical Manual of Mental Disorders (DSM-5-TR), individuals who are formally diagnosed are given a number based on three different functioning levels, which are categorized by the amount of required support. Level 1 autism, often called high-functioning autism, is considered the milder form, and individuals with this diagnosis are noted to "require support." This level also includes that which was once known as Asperger's syndrome, a term which is no longer recognized by the DSM.

The history behind the term Asperger's is downright appalling, as the classification is named after the Austrian physician, Hans Asperger, known for his work alongside Nazi doctors and scientists. A study in Molecular Autism pointed to instances where Asperger referred profoundly disabled children to a clinic that participated in the Third Reich's child euthanasia program that served the Nazi goal of eugenically engineering a genetically 'pure' society through 'racial hygiene' and the elimination of lives deemed a 'burden' and 'not worthy of life' (Czech, 2018).

Levels 2 and 3 are given to those who require "substantial support" and "very substantial support" respectively. What people do not often realize is the subjectivity of these diagnoses due to both the inherent bias of the individual diagnosing as well as the fact that autism is a dynamic disability. When the diagnosed levels of support are determined in the context of assessments, they are subject to the psychologist's personal consideration of "substantial" support.

On top of this, these diagnostic levels are merely a snapshot of the diagnosed individual's functioning at the time of their assessment, which leaves much to be desired for a diagnosis of a dynamic disability.

Level 1-diagnosed autistic individuals are often highly prone to masking and may actually be struggling more internally than their level 3 counterparts. These individuals might be more likely to struggle with shutdown or depression due to their tendency to push through their stress rather than actively working through their symptoms. This is why many autistics prefer "support needs" versus "functioning labels"— these "support needs" can change according to each day or situation the individual finds themselves in. Specific comorbidities can also increase the likelihood of needed support, such as an intellectual disability.

When considering autistic shutdowns or burnout, it is imperative that we understand that no two autistic individuals are exactly the same. Thus, no two shutdowns look the exact same. Sometimes, it's only noted in hindsight that an individual was struggling with a shutdown. It's also not uncommon for instances of shutdown to be misdiagnosed as other disorders, such as depression. While it is very possible for untreated autistic shutdown to lead to depression, an individual can be in shutdown and not be depressed.

When the pandemic hit in 2020, many therapists, myself included, were completely overwhelmed. I was shocked by the sheer number of clients seeking therapy, many for the first time in their lives. I found myself wanting to be around people less and less. This led to my emotions becoming stunted, leading to a deep state of dread. While a part of me feared this might be early signs of depression, I found myself settling on compassion fatigue, which often occurs in those who work in the helping professions. Many times, these professionals appear to either have vicarious symptoms of those they are trying to help, or they start to have physical and emotional symptoms from carrying a consistent heavyweight of helping others without taking care of themselves. At best, this leads to minor negative thoughts regarding one's career of choice. At worst, it brings about doubts as to whether one has the strength to continue in their line of work. Regardless, this phenomenon almost always carries with it feelings of autistic shutdown or long-term burnout.

While I wasn't feeling detached or desiring to leave my line of work, many of the other symptoms were definitely there. I reached out to a local therapist who works with therapists dealing with compassion fatigue—a much-needed specialist in the field. We discussed a great deal about self-care and took some self-inventories that opened my eyes quite a bit. Several sessions in, I mentioned that I was possibly autistic. She noted this, but I don't remember a lot being said on this topic. It wasn't until months after I had started to feel better that I realized in hindsight that what I had wasn't compassion fatigue at all but a clear-cut autistic shutdown. While the treatment was relatively the same and thus rather effective, the difference was rather significant in that I was not consciously aware of what I was dealing with.

Much of this was simply because I was not properly educated on the topic as I should have been— a commonality between myself and many otherwise qualified therapists. The simple understanding of autistic shutdown and the awareness of such a condition may often be the key to prevention and proper treatment. Understanding my brain's predisposition towards overwork and overstimulation has naturally led to an increased ability to combat or prevent autistic shutdowns in advance. Knowing that I am prone to shutdown due to a lack of sleep or an overstimulating sensory environment allows for proper steps to be taken on the front end rather than simply bearing the full brunt of a shutdown episode with no awareness it's even approaching. Knowledge is power! Mindfulness is key! Once you know what a shutdown is and what triggers it for you, you are able to develop tools to better treat or even entirely prevent shutdowns.

LOOKING BACK ON MY FIRST NOTABLE SHUTDOWN

(Trigger warning: Pregnancy loss mentioned)
In 2005, I obtained my first "career job." I was hired as a DCFS caseworker in the foster care unit. This was by far the most demanding job I have ever had due in large part to them being severely understaffed. They needed to double the number of employees in order for the work to adequately be done. I worked there for ten months, but those were the longest ten months of my life. I was working 50-60 hours a week while attending night classes in graduate school.

Exhausted and burned out couldn't cover what I was feeling. I felt that I wasn't the mom I needed to be. How can anyone be with that schedule? Before working at DHS, I worked as a Youth

Care Worker at a residential treatment facility for adolescent sexual offenders. Both of these jobs gave me a lot of insight into the specific traumas of the children that I worked with. It made me a better mother and, eventually a therapist. I even founded and ran a 501(c)3 non-profit for five years to help prevent childhood sexual abuse because of the things I learned. I eventually just combined that program into my counseling.

I was also pregnant with my middle son, Ryker, during a portion of the time I was working at DCFS. I had two back-to-back miscarriages prior to him. I found out I was pregnant with him while at the doctor undergoing testing to find the cause of my miscarriages. The doctor told me that I had super low progesterone and that I was again pregnant and needed to start progesterone treatment immediately, otherwise I would miscarry. Luckily, the treatment worked and Ryker is a miracle because of it. Several months into my pregnancy, I realized that my job was doing more harm than good, so I made the decision to quit.

Looking back on this time, I realize that I pushed through several months of shutdown. I firmly believe that played a part in my hormonal issues and subsequent miscarriages. My mental health also took a hit, and my anxiety was at its peak. I found myself dreading many aspects of my work, but I pushed through because my anxiety would control me if I did not.

Sadly, many individuals get to a point of severe shutdown because they have pushed themselves in their jobs for longer than their bodies and brains could appropriately manage. I did not work for the remaining portion of my pregnancy, and I did not find other work until after I graduated with my degree. I did, however, homeschool my oldest during a portion of his kindergarten year. There is no way I could have appropriately managed a new baby, homeschooling, parenting three children, and the rest of my graduate classes in a reasonable manner.

CHAPTER THREE

WHEN SHUTDOWNS LEAD TO MELTDOWNS

Yes, adults can have meltdowns— even some allistic ones. Many autistic adults have meltdowns, which may look vastly different from person to person. It's no surprise that when individuals face more overwhelming situations than they can handle, meltdowns may occur as a result. Unfortunately, these meltdowns may lead to such intense negative emotions that autistic individuals are often predisposed to self-harming or suicidal behaviors. These behaviors are incredibly destructive on their own, but they often carry with them intense feelings of embarrassment, shame, and guilt. I know these feelings all too well.

While meltdowns can occur outside of an episode of shutdown, it is important for individuals in the midst of a shutdown episode to understand that they are more vulnerable to meltdowns. Similar to the neurology behind shutdowns, the PFC (prefrontal cortex) is heavily affected during a meltdown. This area of the brain is the most integral part of our brain in regulating emotions and impulses. Under normal conditions, this part of the brain is a powerhouse that allows us to think rationally and perform as needed. Under intense stress, however, the prefrontal cortex is easily overpowered by other less calculating parts of the brain. During a shutdown, the performance of our prefrontal cortex is hindered by acute stress, thus leaving a clear path for emotional dysregulation to take over, which often leads to behaviors indicative of a meltdown.

Emotional dysregulation occurs when we are unable to manage our emotions. This often occurs when our nervous system has "perceived" a threat of some kind and goes into a fight, flight, freeze, or fawn response. These emotions may often appear to be out of context in comparison to the situation that provoked them. This dysregulation can often take us outside of our window of tolerance, which is the state of being in which we are able to manage our emotions and not be overwhelmed by stress (Pedersen, 2022). Emotional dysregulation is seen in many conditions and disorders, but due to their particular brain chemistry, autistics are more apt to become emotionally dysregulated more frequently.

There is a great deal of neurology behind a meltdown. According to research from Arnsten et al. (2012), during episodes of stress, our brain floods with the arousal chemicals noradrenaline and dopamine, signaling the PFC to shut off neuron firing, which results in diminishing network activity and our ability to regulate behavior. Self-control is even more affected during this process because the hypothalamus has sent signals to the adrenal glands near the kidneys to release cortisol into the bloodstream, which goes back to the brain and causes the neurons in the PFC to stop firing (Arnsten et al., 2012). The more primitive parts of the brain are, therefore, taking control, including the amygdala, which is our alerting network to our nervous system.

Biologically, these processes make sense if we are indeed under a real threat. I am certain they were extremely important in days when threats were everywhere, and we were at risk of becoming food sources for another apex predator. However, our brains have not received the memo that we have evolved past that point. Autistic meltdowns occur when these internal processes coded for survival are triggered by overstimulation or high anxiety. Examples of such triggering events may include not being able to remove oneself from a bustling environment, being unprepared for a change, or having a disagreement. The wear and tear these processes have on an individual builds up over time during a shutdown, and it may be something seemingly minor that ends up sending them over the edge.

The behaviors exhibited during a meltdown can look vastly different. They can range from behaviors as simple as crying or sobbing to more aggressive behaviors such as hitting oneself or others, kicking, biting, pulling out hair, screaming, yelling, or intense stimming such as rocking or humming. This large spectrum of behaviors is due to the areas of the brain that trigger the fight, flight, freeze, or fawn response. It's not uncommon at all for an individual to respond with a fighting behavior followed by a fleeing of some type, such as running away. And yes, I am still talking about adults. While we definitely see these behaviors in children, it isn't uncommon for an autistic adult to also display these behaviors. Yet, we are more apt to criticize these behaviors when displayed by an adult versus a child.

A classic example of a meltdown manifested by an overwhelmed individual was demonstrated perfectly on screen in the movie Shrek Forever After (2010). The scene called "Do the Roar" included an already over-it Shrek being bombarded by a barrage of overstimulating noises and prods while being asked to roar, get the cake while not forgetting the candles, keep Donkey away from the said cake, roar again, then get accused of licking the cake and forgetting the candles, then be told to watch cake only for the three pigs to eat it in a split second, then go straight to trying to calm his babies, while Pinocchio runs circles around him at a fast speed.

Shrek inevitably breaks down and gives a very loud roar, followed by applause from everyone. When another cake is presented by Puss in Boots, Fiona finally notices that Shrek is not doing okay and checks in on him. It is too late, however, and Shrek goes full Hulk smash into the new cake. He then leaves the party, much to the shock of all the party attendees. I was overwhelmed two seconds into that scene and would have snapped a lot sooner. For many autistics, that is what overstimulation that leads to meltdowns feels like, but the triggers can be much smaller.

I have personally noted a vast array of symptoms described to me by my clients during their meltdowns, including symptoms of dissociation. Some have reported intense confusion to the point where they are not sure where they are, and nothing makes sense to them. Others have described feelings of intense derealization or depersonalization. This occurs when an individual feels either like the events occurring are not real or that they are a spectator rather than an active participant in the events unfolding. While the specific neural functions of dissociation are ambiguous in nature, it is not that hard to imagine these symptoms occurring during a meltdown, considering all that is going on in the brain and in the PFC.

It is important to understand that meltdowns are not temper tantrums. It is understandable how these can get confused in children, but even with them, once you have a basic understanding of the premise and reasoning behind both, they are easy to differentiate. Tantrums are manipulative in nature. They are meant as a means to try and control a person's behavior or get something in return. They are goal-oriented. This can be the child in the checkout line screaming his head off because he wants candy or the boss yelling and screaming at his employees to work harder. While it may be a few minutes or so before these individuals can get back to a baseline emotional state, their behavior is driven by a goal, and the behavior dissipates upon achieving that goal.

Typically, I describe meltdowns as runaway trains. No amount of getting their way — despite what they are saying — will get them back to a baseline emotional state quickly. The train just needs to derail or come to its own stopping point. Think of the child exhausted from no nap, screaming her head off for her teddy bear, but if someone hands her the teddy bear she still screams and throws it. This is meltdown territory brought on by a lack of sleep as a primary trigger. Even as an adult, I find this trigger to be my biggest one.

According to Maslow's hierarchy of needs, physiological needs are the primary needs that must be met before an individual can attend to the higher order of needs. In my case, that primary need is sleep. If I am sleep-deprived, I am not even concerned about hunger, thirst, or where I lay my head down. My need for sleep is at the forefront of my mind. My biology has also shown that my brain rebels into the risk of seizures if I am deprived for too long, so I do all I can to mitigate this risk and minimize this as a trigger to my meltdowns.

It is imperative for all individuals to understand the intensity behind a meltdown. An individual can have a normal, healthy crying episode and not fall into meltdown territory. I have always said as a therapist that crying is one of the most natural coping mechanisms we have built in us. Research has shown that tears have the capacity to offer health benefits by releasing oxytocin and endogenous opioids, also known as endorphins or feel-good chemicals, which can help ease both physical and emotional pain (Newhouse, 2021). Meltdown crying is vastly different. It is extremely intense, overwhelming, and often flooded with negative thoughts.

When I would have these intense bouts of meltdown crying as a child, it would be accompanied by what I now know to be "double breathing." My father referred to this as "huffing" and would get angry when I wouldn't stop doing it, but he obviously didn't understand the physiology behind it. And for the record, I hold no ill feelings towards my parents for their reactions. Sadly, this was not an uncommon reaction from parents of the eighties who were very ignorant of the science behind meltdowns versus tantrums.

Double breathing is a symptom of acute hyperventilation that occurs during intense emotional distress, such as meltdown, crying or panic attacks. Intense crying can often create a disturbance in the regular respiratory function of the lungs and diaphragm, which can force the diaphragm out of rhythm, preventing blood oxygen and carbon dioxide levels from remaining consistent (O'Connor, 2021). Sadly, my father's reaction worsened my double breathing. If you or someone you know is actively double breathing, try finding a paper bag to breathe in or follow a model of breathing that requires slow inhales and almost twice as long exhales. There are also a lot of great free phone apps out there that can help with breathing exercises. I enjoy the ones where I can have a visualization guiding my inhales and exhales.

Panic attacks and meltdowns are not the same. However, a panic attack can follow a meltdown. This is what was happening to me as a child. While the neurology may begin similarly to that of a meltdown at first, another stress hormone called norepinephrine is also released during a panic attack. The release of this hormone causes a spike in the person's heart rate and blood pressure, leading to the person experiencing overwhelming dread and panic (Bruning, 2018). Panic attacks also take a significantly longer time to abate, sometimes up to three days.

Many individuals find themselves in emergency rooms because of the fear that they are having a heart attack. Mindfulness, meditation, and breathing exercises can often help the panic attack subside. Some individuals are prescribed medications to help cope with a panic disorder. It is important to understand that many doctors are often reluctant to prescribe medications because of the tendency for many of these medications to be highly addictive. If one's panic attacks can be reduced with positive coping techniques, they are preferable to medications. Positive coping techniques are more likely to reduce panic attacks from coming on in the first place as they teach how to monitor one's bodily reactions to stimuli and triggers and practice them as a preventive measure.

Meltdowns may come on slower than panic attacks, but the intensity behind them can be just as frightening. The individual experiencing the meltdown can be at acute risk of self-harm. Because the PFC is the area of the brain being affected the most, the individual is at risk of acting more impulsively. Meltdowns can be exacerbated by the multitude of negative thoughts that seem to occur during an episode. These episodes feel so intense and so awful that the individual just wants them to stop.

Outside of the depression I experienced in early adulthood, I don't struggle with suicidal thoughts unless I am actively having a meltdown. I didn't recognize this pattern until a couple of years ago. Before making the connection between my meltdowns and suicidal thoughts, I was always left confused following my meltdowns. I would wonder if I was depressed since professionals in the mental health field generally agree that being suicidal indicates depression. As was the case with me, however, this sentiment is not entirely accurate.

I am generally content with my life and have been for most of it. I had one major depressive episode at eighteen and a couple of mild ones over the years that I took an active role in preventing from getting worse. Even in those mild ones, I did not have suicidal thoughts because there were no meltdowns during that time. While my meltdowns are infrequent, the intensity and awfulness are equated to that of an extremely heavy sorrow mixed with shame and guilt. I just want the feeling to go away. I want to not feel like a burden, which is often one of the most common awful negative thoughts that occur during these episodes for me. Sometimes, these thoughts are spoken out loud, but most of the time, they are internal. My husband has been the only individual to hear me speak to them, and that has only been recently when I deliberately share my vulnerability with him.

I have heard the same thoughts from others, though. According to many clients, this is a common issue during the midst of an episode. This is not just an issue with adults either. I see it with children and teens as well. This can cause other situational stressors because if the environment that a child is in when they make these statements is not neurodiversity informed, they can actually do things to make the situation worse.

Acute hospital settings are often not the most ideal for many autistic children or adults. They are the absolute worst sensory environment and are often more likely to cause more traumatic reactions. I worked at an acute hospital during my graduate school internship and my first therapist position. There is a time and need for those places, but meltdowns are not those times. However, because many schools and hospitals immediately assume suicidal ideation (SI) is something to be assessed, that is their immediate reaction.

Coping With Meltdowns

Despite the intensity and awfulness that is a meltdown, one must realize that they are indeed temporary. Now that I am aware of what is happening in my brain, I practice mindfulness to help me get through them. I tell myself that I will not feel like this tomorrow, that it just feels awful right now, and that I will get through this. When my husband was present during one, he was able to remind me of this as well.

Supporting a loved one is the absolute best way to help them cope with a meltdown. Remind them that they are loved and that you are there with them. Tell them it is okay to feel whatever they are feeling but remind them that those feelings will subside. Whatever you do, DO NOT guilt or shame them. You will most likely make it worse and increase the likelihood that they will try to impulsively harm themselves. Shame spirals occur when an individual cannot escape the negative thoughts, which can lead to more intense dangerous thoughts.

Try to get to the safest environment that you can during a meltdown. This might be a sensory room if you are one of the rare few who have them, or it can be your bedroom on your bed. Grounding techniques can often be helpful, but during a flipped amygdala, it is often difficult to focus on identifying things to touch, taste, hear, see, or smell. Something I recommend to many clients in the midst of a panic attack and a meltdown is what I call a shock grounding technique. Shock because it uses all of your senses at once, regardless of whether you want it to or not.

This intervention requires a whole lemon. Bite into the lemon, rind and all, and then spit it out. In doing this, all of your senses have been shocked in that split second. You see the yellow lemon; note the color. It's hard not to. You touch the lemon and feel the grainy texture of the rind. Biting into the lemon, you hear the crunch. You feel the hardness of the rind contrasting with the softness of the lemon's flesh in your mouth. You smell the lemon's pungent scent and taste its bitter sourness. In one quick motion, you have ignited all of your senses. A lemon is ideal because the shock of the sour adds to the grounding effect; however, if you are really opposed to lemons, my next suggestion would be an orange or a lime. I have even had clients use salt. Whatever works for you, use it, so long as it isn't harmful.

This technique has been known to stop a panic attack in its tracks better than many addictive medications can. It can also be used in the midst of a meltdown to ground your thoughts. Practicing mindful deep breathing, as described earlier, is also useful. This deep breathing gets more oxygen to the brain and activates the parasympathetic nervous system, which sends a signal to your brain to tell the PFC that you're safe and you don't need to use the fight, flight, freeze, or fawn response.

Other means to cope with a meltdown include utilizing your stims. Stims are self-regulatory behaviors that can help manage over or under-stimulation, emotions, and pain. They are not just something autistics use. Many allistic and neurotypical individuals use them as well. The most frequently used stims include leg bouncing, nail-biting, and humming. Echolalia, hand flapping, bouncing, and spinning can be common stims for autistics.

My daughter bounces on a ball or jumps on a mini trampoline while humming as a primary stim, both when she is happy and when she is upset. Humming is a very healthy stim. According to a blog in Flowly (2022), humming greatly increases nasal nitric oxide, a neural transmitter that is released as a gas to sterilize the air you breathe, protecting your body by sterilizing airborne pathogens. It can also help stimulate your vagus nerve, a key role in activating the parasympathetic nervous system, otherwise known as your "rest and digest" state, and improve heart rate variability.

We should never try to remove healthy stims from an autistic individual's coping toolkit.

To determine if a stim is healthy, there are four questions you can ask. These are also the same questions to determine if a coping skill is healthy:

1. Is it easy to do?
2. Is it good for you?
3. Is it good for others?
4. Does it make you feel good?

I learned these four questions during my training to become a play therapist; however, they are useful for all ages, not just children, especially since adults are typically the most likely to utilize an unhealthy coping mechanism. If the answer to all of these questions is yes, then the individual should be allowed to use it. If not, redirect to a stim that does fit. If it's distracting others but needed at a specific time, provide a space and time for the individual to use it. This is typically something that might occur during a school environment. An individual having a meltdown should be brought to a private, quiet space anyways, so distracting others shouldn't even be an issue.

It wasn't until last year that I made the discovery that deep pressure and hugs are some of the best supports for me during a meltdown. Sadly, for most of my life, I was alone as I tried to hide away during meltdowns. In the few times they were in front of others, I was not given this simple support because many do not know of its strong healing power. My husband held me during one of my worst ones, and while it didn't stop the meltdown immediately, I found it reduced the negative thoughts first. It made sense, considering this is what we ideally try to do when my daughter is having a meltdown.

Not all autistics prefer pressure or hugs. There are some that are averse to touch in general. This should be respected. But you can still be a big support for these individuals by just being present and reassuring them throughout. Even if they ask for space, tell them you are nearby if they need anything. Comfort and support are key. I just wish I would have figured this out many years ago.

Recouping From a Meltdown

Meltdowns are extremely emotionally and physically draining. They will likely lead to increased burnout and shutdown, even if you weren't in one prior to the meltdown. The sheer exhaustion of intense ones can mimic that of an extreme workout. I played roller derby for the five years between my third and fourth child. It was a big, focused interest of mine at the time. I was a jammer, which is the person skating around the pack at a more intense pace, scoring points, and being knocked all kinds of ways by the blockers of the opposing team. Every morning after the day of a bout, I would wake up extremely physically exhausted and unable to move very well. Every time I have had an intense meltdown, I would wake up the next day feeling worse than this because I am not only physically depleted but also emotionally beaten down. Meltdown recovery is no joke.

It is inevitable that many autistics will have intense guilt and shame spirals after a meltdown, which is why the emotional state is so affected. The days following a meltdown can mimic signs of major depression. Many individuals find it difficult to leave their bed or home, and their motivation to do things is very low. Hygiene and appetite are very likely to be affected. If one is able to take a day or two off work, that can be a great help in recovering. If you can manage to have low or no demands at all, even better. You can call this the mental flu if you need to.

Much like the acute time after a meltdown, loved ones and supportive figures are most needed during this time by just being present and offering assistance if necessary. And again, refrain from guilting and shaming them. They are still highly vulnerable during this time. There are also some autistics who feel as if their meltdowns are a good reset for them. Perhaps it's the buildup of everything that has been consuming them for a while that is no longer a burden to them. For them, the buildup might have been more uncomfortable than the actual meltdown, and now that the weight is lifted, they can begin to move again.

THE MELTDOWN THAT LED TO MY DIAGNOSIS

It was the end of 2019 when I began my second private practice, which consisted of neurodiversity-affirming group counseling and consulting. I also started an MBA in early 2020 and completed it at the end of 2021. It was during those two years that the pandemic hit. When 2022 came around, my goal was to simply try to rest and restore. But as usual, life had other plans.

My oldest daughter, Kieran, got engaged in November of 2021. This was not a huge surprise as she had been with her boyfriend for three years, and they had been clear about their intentions for some time. But with an actual engagement comes actual planning, and we had eight months until they wanted to get married. I should also point out that this was her senior year of high school, so we were still in the depths of getting all of her senior-year things done, such as applying for college, finding scholarships, and taking senior pictures (which I did myself).

Each month brought about new things and new changes. While these were mostly good changes, change in general is difficult to adjust to as an autistic adult. My oldest, Gage, found a job and decided he wanted to start looking for his own place, which was something we had been pushing toward for some time. I was also in the midst of planning a beach vacation for the whole family that upcoming summer. The first half of the year consisted of a lot of logistical and planning stress and not much rest.

With all the wedding planning, there came double empathy struggles and arguments with my daughter. I was also struggling with the fact that her 18th year planning a wedding was also reminiscent of my 18th year, which — if you will remember — was the most traumatic year of my life. I tried to be open about that, but I do not think my family quite understood where my head was at with all this, and I was not the best at being able to express this at the time.

Everything came to a head one evening during a particular argument that got very heated, and my husband made the mistake of trying to shut us both down completely. I tried to explain that I needed to be heard and that I was trying to come from a place of empathy, but he would not let me talk at all. This quickly escalated to one of the worst meltdowns I have ever had as an adult and was reminiscent of the ones I had as a child when no one was around. Ones where I would scream, cry, hit my head, run away from situations, etc. This was also several months into various conversations with him about my opening up more about my self-realized autism and how certain things affect me, especially demands and being controlled.

One such thing that I had been incredibly open about was my Pathological Demand Avoidance (PDA) and how it strikes a fight response rather than one of flight or freeze. I felt as if he had simply forgotten everything I tried to tell him. I felt trapped. I felt unheard. I felt everything that was awful in those brief moments.

The following days involved a forced emotional shutdown mixed with intense guilt and shame. I barely left my bedroom. I did not eat. I felt broken and lost. And despite my exhaustion, both mentally and physically, I was not able to sleep much. Luckily for me, this was on the weekend, and I was not supposed to be anywhere. Otherwise, I am not certain how I would have functioned. When I started making myself come out, I could barely talk to anyone without tears welling up. This was unlike me, as I normally struggle to make myself cry even when I need to. I felt extremely broken and vulnerable.

One by one, I approached those who were affected and expressed myself the best way I could. While I apologized for my behavior, I emphasized to my husband that I had trusted that he knew better after trying to express myself previously. I told him I felt hurt that he disregarded my vulnerability in telling him my struggles only to do the one thing that could bring out the worst response in me. I found it all especially odd considering in 25 years together, he had never once done that before. I then informed him that I made the decision to get formally evaluated because I didn't feel that he would take me seriously otherwise. I also apologized to my daughter and told her the same about my decision to get tested. Little by little, I tried to move forward, but it was extremely difficult.

Unfortunately, the path to getting a formal diagnosis is not an easy one for many. It is definitely a privilege, with a lot of gatekeeping in the way, which is why self-diagnosis is considered valid in much of the autism community. It saddens me when I hear some autistics or allistics are very opposed to acknowledging self-diagnoses. For one, the number of Psychologists who offer testing to adults who may have autism is very few. Even in our area, there are only a handful, and those who test and diagnose adults only accept certain insurance policies. If you are an adult with Medicaid in Arkansas, there are very few psychologists who accept it—the same is true in many other states. At the time of my diagnosis, there were none in Northwest Arkansas. If you are willing to pay out of pocket for testing, the bill comes to anywhere between $1000-$2000. Even when one is tested, many evaluators use outdated and often ableist testing measures created to diagnose young children. Of the few in the area whom I trusted, most knew of me through my referrals. Thus, I feared bias, though probably unnecessarily.

I looked further outside of our area and found one in another state that utilized up-to-date testing measures and had appropriate language on their site about understanding high masking autism in adults. She did not accept insurance, however, and it would be a long drive for testing. But I was willing, and thanks to PsyPact, I would be able to do it. I should also note the cost quoted to me was above the average cost I listed in the previous paragraph. When I reached out to schedule, like most places, there was a wait of six months, which is another hurdle to many. I went ahead and scheduled and completed all the intake paperwork. Once that was set, there was a bit of relief but also increased ambivalence.

In the meantime, life continued to be remarkably busy, and I was over the top stressed with everything. Kieran later graduated with honors and with a year of college classes already under her belt. Wedding plans were all soon finalized, and the day of her wedding was busy from sunup to sundown. Everything went beautifully, and I managed well with the stress given I had a ton of help from the groomsmen, bridesmaids, and family. I went directly from planning for a wedding to a vacation as the plan was for them to return from their honeymoon in Portland, OR, to then leave soon after with us to Galveston, TX.

On the day of our departure, five minutes before we were set to leave, two neighbor dogs broke through a fence in our backyard and attacked one of our dogs, severely maiming her. I was the first to notice Harley was covered in blood. I screamed and went into freakout mode. What followed was a blur of an emergency vet visit, talks with police, and logistical changes. My mother was set to watch the house and our dogs. We left hours later than planned, with the initial news from the vet to be somewhat positive.

It was not until we nearly reached our destination that we were given grim news. It would be unlikely she would make it, and she was in extreme pain even with the maximum amount of pain medication they could give her. We made the only decision we felt we could and had to say our goodbyes from far away. My mother got to be with her in person. The rest of the vacation was marred by this awful trauma. It broke us all at various times during the trip.

On our way home, we had just broken off from Kieran and her husband, who were going to visit his family, when we started to note the signs of our van breaking down. I was driving and pulled off near the spot of an old, closed gas station in the middle of nowhere Oklahoma in the intense heat of summer. I remember barely making it to a good spot when it completely died. I stepped out of the van and put my head between my knees, knowing this was not good. My husband had no service, and I had just a few bars on our cell phones. I made attempts at calling for a tow, and there were none local. I was feeling desperate and scared. I had four of my children with me, and we were nowhere close to anything. I remember thinking, "This is how horror movies start." I should know, as they are my favorite movie genre.

When we had no luck getting a tow, we made the decision to start calling family. All our family lived in Oklahoma, but not near there. Steven's parents and one of his brothers rallied some forces and drove all the way to us with a tow truck and lent us a vehicle to get home the rest of the way while they took our van with them to get fixed. While we waited for them to get there, my mother-in-law made a call to a local church that allowed us to stay in from the heat and gave us some food. I cannot thank them enough for their kindness and generosity. What could have been a disastrous event ended up being okay despite the amount of stress we were under.

We made it home in the early hours of the morning, with my mother still waiting. We were drained and mentally exhausted, and I was teetering on the edge of total shutdown. Luckily, I had carved out some days prior to having to return to work, all of which I used to try and decompress as much as I possibly could. I honestly could have used an extra day or two.

It was around this time that I had a check-in with a former client and received word on a new Psychologist in the area that was offering testing for adults with autism. This client had a pleasant experience, and it sounded similar to the needs of my own, so I decided to reach out for myself since there was no fear of bias, having not referred to them prior. Not only were they able to take my insurance, but they were able to get me in within the month. This would be three months sooner than my scheduled appointment with the other Psychologist in the next state. I took that spot and immediately felt a sense of relief and hope. I went ahead and asked to be evaluated for autism and ADHD as just a rule out since there are symptoms that overlap.

I spent the next few weeks writing up my history since I am more expressively written than I am verbal. My fear was that I would forget all the things in my childhood and adult life that were signs, and then I would not get a thorough view of things. My husband also agreed to do an informant interview or test if needed. I had two appointments for my testing, not including the appointment to review the results. It was about six weeks between the first interview and the results interview. There were nine different assessments, including the clinical interview and the one my husband completed. The ones that I felt asked the right questions for me were the Social Responsiveness Scale-2nd Edition Adult and the Sensory Profile 2.

The waiting between the assessments and the results was difficult. There was a lot of imposter syndrome setting in. Doubts and questions about maybe the intelligence test will come back and show I am deficient, and that is the reason for everything. Or thoughts that the Personality Assessment Inventory (PAI) will show something I never even had a clue about. Fears that I had never even considered were popping up. That honestly should have been a blaring red flag there to me about my tendency to overanalyze things.

The day of the results came, and I was a ball of nerves. I made the mistake of scheduling my own sessions immediately, not allowing for any time to process things if needed. Finally, I was given a diagnosis of Autism Spectrum Disorder and Generalized Anxiety Disorder. ADHD was ruled out, and the Psychologist stated that that assessment was one of the cleanest she had ever seen and that the symptoms that I did have of ADHD were ones that overlapped with both. I will point out that it is definitely possible for an individual to have both, but for me, my symptoms just align with autism.

So here it was. The finality of it all. Answers in hand. Luckily, nothing major surprising came about, and I did not need the time to process what I feared I would need. My husband bought me a cake and scrawled "Congrats on your Autism" on it. I sent this out to my family, and this is how I told them my results. I got laughs and no pushback. I would like to think this had something to do with the fact I was super open and honest about things and had been taking my mask off for the past few months. My daughter had even used this picture of my cake as part of one of her presentation assignments at her college when she discussed neurodiversity. Come to find out the professor opened up about being autistic and ADHD and enjoyed seeing this side of things being out in the open. That right there is the reason I am now a lot more open about who I am—Because I know I am not alone.

CHAPTER FOUR

MASKING

M asking is one of the most difficult things to unlearn as an adult. I have done this mostly unconsciously my whole life. While I was sometimes aware that I was making a change in my behavior to meet the norm, I honestly thought that everyone did that. But just in case my assumption was wrong, I never let on to the fact that I was playing a role. I felt as if I was switching characters to fit whatever a certain situation or setting required of me.

Instances of me masking stretch back as far as I can remember. Even in kindergarten, raising a hand to be called on was an unspoken rule that I had yet to be made aware of. Despite not understanding this concept, I raised my hand along with everybody else when my teacher asked a question. Thank goodness I wasn't called on. Otherwise, I would sharply remember the embarrassment.

An incident where my attempt at masking did not go as smoothly occurred in first grade. My teacher went around and asked everyone if they were male or female, and I was unfamiliar with these terms. While I was generally good at identifying patterns and adjusting my behaviors accordingly, I struggled to identify the pattern in this instance. I paid attention to each kid's answer to try and determine what my own would be, and I noticed that all of my friends responded that they were male. Thus, when it was my turn to answer, I answered that I was male. I was quickly corrected by the teacher before she moved on to the next person. I internally shrugged and thought nothing of it, still not understanding the difference.

Abstract and conceptual thinking can be difficult for autistic individuals of all ages. This is why many autistics are very literal. Unspoken rules are especially challenging as it can be a struggle to read between the lines. Autistics prefer concrete explanations and dislike vague ones. Sarcasm is also rather perplexing to autistics, which is a personal struggle as an autistic adult married to an individual whose primary language is sarcasm.

My husband is a teacher and has expressed at times how his sarcasm has fallen short on certain students. I have made him aware of how autistic teens will often struggle with that, and luckily, he has realized that his sarcasm can be seen as too abstract for them. Sarcasm isn't the only way teachers can be too vague. If you are a teacher, please be aware that you must be as concrete as possible in all your interactions with students (Moreno & O'Neal, 2000). Don't leave it up to them to read between the lines.

Oftentimes, autistic's attempts at fitting neurotypical behavior can fall short. The most common places for this to occur are in the classroom, work environment, and social situations. That's pretty much the accumulation of everything outside of the home. An autistic's home space may be the only place where they feel free to be themselves, given how exhausting masking is.

WHAT IS MASKING?

According to an article from the National Autistic Society and Dr. Hannah Belcher (2022), masking involves the suppression of certain behaviors that one finds soothing but might not fit the "norm," such as stimming or intense interests. It can also include mimicking or changing our behaviors to match those around us (also known as code-switching), developing complex social scripts to get through social situations, and copying non-verbal behaviors (Belcher, 2022). In essence, the goal of masking is to hide one's true self, be it intentionally or unintentionally, as a social survival strategy.

Specific masking behaviors include, but are not limited to, forcing eye contact during conversations, hiding personal interests, scripting conversations, pushing through intense sensory environments, disguising stimming behaviors, mimicking facial gestures, and imitating other non-verbal behaviors (Stanborough, 2021). Eye contact seems to be a rather difficult one for many autistics. Some cannot mask it and avoid it completely. I find that it's only in certain situations that I find it rather difficult.

I can maintain eye contact with those close to me with little to no effort. During one-on-one sessions with clients, I also find it not very difficult; however, I am certain I look away quite often but do so in what I believe to be a very natural way. However, I cannot do it in passing, in crowds, or to those I meet with briefly, such as in a drive-through. It is almost painful but definitely uncomfortable. It is also something I find has actually gotten more difficult the older I get.

Scripting is a common thing done in our household. Not necessarily as a means to mask but as a fun, jovial way to interact. We script or quote movies, cartoons, or just about anything we have found to be humorous. However, when scripting is done as a means to mask, it is not fun. Scripting is a form of delayed echolalia that has communicative intent. If an individual makes changes in wording or intonation made by the original speaker, it is considered mitigated echolalia, which is a more advanced form of scripting (Fox, 2019).

I remember a clear incident of scripting I used when I was about to leave for the NAVY at the Military Entrance Processing Station (MEPS). The night prior at the hotel, I talked with no one except my roommate, despite several attempts by the males who were also there. I wasn't masking my displeasure at all at one point when I was trying to make a call to my husband, who was my boyfriend at the time, and some were trying very rudely to interrupt me. I made clear eye rolls and turned my back to them, before ending my call and going back to my room.

Before getting on the plane the next day, there were some last-minute things we had to go through at the MEPS, which took several hours. At one point, I had to be driven in a taxi across town to get my left eye tested by an eye doctor. When I returned, lunch was just about over. Most had already left the lunch area, and there was just one table with three guys at it. I remember thinking I would prefer to sit alone but that I look pathetic. Putting on my bravest mask, I walked up to them and asked if the one empty chair had been taken.

The scripted words were something I had seen many times on TV, yet they fit the situation perfectly. That didn't seem abnormal to me, but this is one of many situations in which I have used stuff from TV to start a conversation. I remember their faces though. They looked shocked and told me I could sit. These were complete strangers to me, but I made it work and actually spent the rest of my time there talking with them before heading out. Scripting helped me find a group to blend in with. However, it was still exhausting to do. This interaction also included aspects of code-switching because I manipulated my own behavior to appeal to this group, which is something that I do on a regular basis.

Code-switching has been something that has come relatively easily to me. From a young age, even if I didn't understand the reasoning behind behaviors, I was able to identify patterns in the typical behaviors of others and match them as needed. As time went on, this skill evolved to the point where I was able to pick up on incongruences between people's verbal communication and non-verbal behaviors. For example, while someone might tell me that they are doing fine, my internal response may indicate otherwise based on their behaviors. Noticing these mismatched patterns of behavior triggers an autonomic response causing my mood to change. This ability has become a valuable skill to have as a therapist and as a parent, but it also has its downsides because along with high somatic empathy comes a hyper-awareness which can be draining emotionally and physically over time.

Pushing through overstimulating sensory environments is another common mask, and it is one that probably depletes my battery faster than anything. I really wish noise-canceling headphones were as common in the '80s and '90s as they are today. They are one of my most common IEP or 504 recommendations. While loud environments as a whole are difficult for me, I find that pushing through situations that trigger misophonia, or difficult emotional responses to certain noises, are especially draining. Sharing rooms with those who snore ignites a visceral anger response in me. Loud base in vehicles is another misophonic anger trigger. I used to have a friend in high school that I could hear coming for several minutes before he would arrive, and I would cringe every time. He found humor during the times I had to ride with him as I would sit with my hands covering my ears. Instead of turning it down, he would just torture me further, finding amusement in my misery. Looking back, that should have been a red flag about that individual. I still flinch when I hear base in vehicles. I literally believe I can feel it in my bones.

Masking through loud sensory environments is perhaps one of the biggest triggers many students and employees have that will lead to shutdowns and meltdowns. I have no doubt in my mind that this was one of the primary triggers of my daughter's meltdowns at school before we ended up taking her out to homeschool. Schools can be extremely loud environments, and no number of noise-canceling headphones can block that out. During her last year in public school, my daughter was struggling with the sensory pain of wearing headphones. Therefore, she wasn't wearing them even when she needed to.

I personally struggle with wearing headphones and earpieces for too long as well, so it is a complicated sensory struggle for me at times. When I go out to eat, I typically have to wear my Loop earplugs if the restaurant is loud at all. Cracker Barrell is the absolute worst! By the time I take them out, though, my ears are hurting. I couldn't imagine having to wear them for too long.

For those in work environments that are triggering, finding ways to accommodate their needs can be a rather difficult endeavor. Many places refuse to make accommodations unless you have a specific diagnosis, and even then, they want it spelled out by a professional, so self-diagnosed individuals are pretty much out of luck. I have had clients go through formal testing just to get the diagnosis to be able to succeed at work. This is ableist, and if you are a leader or a boss that requires this, please stop.

Many corporate environments are shifting to a more open community layout, believing this will drive teamwork. I cannot stress enough how this is the worst environment for an autistic with sensory sensitivities. Fast-paced environments such as fast food are another work environment that can be problematic for the sensory sensitive. Many times, these environments will lead an individual to cope by masking for fear of getting fired.

Even some remote positions require cameras to be on constantly, and to an autistic individual, this can feel the same as having a supervisor stand in front of you all day, expecting regular eye contact. I don't even think many allistics would appreciate that, but that is what an autistic feels with continuous camera monitoring. Trying to get the company to allow the accommodation of no camera monitoring is often seen as a want and not a need despite it affecting neither the company financially nor any of the employee's job duties. If the autistic individual is forced to mask through this, it will inevitably lead to less focus and high anxiety which is not good for the company or the employee. A simple accommodation of routine camera check-ins versus continuous monitoring can make all the difference.

While both genders are capable of masking, research has shown that individuals who identify as women are more likely to camouflage or mask their autism than those who identify as men (Hull et al., 2019). This is also why many women are not diagnosed until much later in life, such as I was. This delay can often exasperate mental health issues because of the lack of support these individuals receive. According to research, nearly 80% of autistic women are often misdiagnosed with conditions such as borderline personality disorder, bipolar disorder, eating disorders, and anxiety (McCrossin, 2022). While there certainly can be these comorbidities, autism as a primary diagnosis is often missed.

Research has been consistently clear that the effects of masking are detrimental to one's mental health. While it may be beneficial at times to help navigate through various social situations, it is also clear that it is a very taxing and exhausting maladaptive behavior that leads to increased stress, anxiety, depression, exhaustion, and suicidality (Cage & Troxell-Whitman, 2019). It also leads to individuals losing their sense of identity. This is one aspect I was not quite prepared for when I did get my official diagnosis. I had to look back and review my whole life through a different lens. I questioned who I even was, where I began, and where my mask ended. This is still a process of trying to unlearn to unmask. Luckily, there are some resources out there that I have found to be helpful, including books from other late-diagnosed autistics (see the resources section for some of these books).

It is evident how masking can and will lead to shutdowns. Even those who are not typically high-masking are still at high risk for them. My daughter is a classic example of this. I have always envied her ability to just be herself. She was given the most free-spirited award in preschool, and that is definitely her. She doesn't care how she is perceived and does things her own way despite what others tell her to. However, she still gets to points that I recognize are shutdowns. I am pretty certain that is what was happening before I took her out of public school. The demands of everything were still getting to her, and she wasn't even trying to mask it.

ACKNOWLEDGING MY MASK AND MY DIAGNOSIS

My youngest, Ridlee, was born at home in January 2014. She was diagnosed with autism at the age of 4 years old. Initially, we thought she had Pragmatic Communication Disorder. No other signs stuck out that seemed to be off to me. That would later be a red flag indicator for me for my own neurology.

It was during her assessment with the psychologist that he began asking me specific questions that I noted were things I did as a child or things that I still do on occasion. Many of these things were not always done in front of others because they were things I enjoyed doing when I was alone. Other such things were your typical things, such as brief eye contact. He noted she made very brief eye contact. But so do I. Why does one have to look for extended periods at people's faces? That has never felt comfortable for me. If I am in drive-thrus, I will not look at their faces at all; however, no one had ever seemed bothered by that, so why was it an issue? In short, I left with more questions about myself than I had answers about Ridlee that day. She was formally diagnosed with Autism Spectrum Disorder following that appointment, thus planting the seed that I, too, might be autistic because she is like me in many ways. The only difference between us is that she does not hide or mask her symptoms.

After her diagnosis, I delved deep into the topic of autism. I read books, articles, and blogs that eventually led me to autistic-led groups on social media platforms. The autistic community is where I was learning the most. This focused interest is not something out of character for me. After receiving my full licensure, I delved into several different specialties and accumulated various certifications and licenses in substance misuse, addiction, and play therapy.

Once something grabs my interest, I bury myself in learning as much about it as I possibly can. Autism and neurodiversity just became my new focused interest, but because this topic was hitting closer to home for me, I dug into it like never before. The more I dug, the more I would see myself in many late-diagnosed autistic adults, particularly that of high-masking females. I began identifying as self-realized or self-diagnosed about two years after my daughter's diagnosis. I kept this mostly to myself and only discussed it with my husband for a while.

Occasionally, I would make statements about my daughter and me being a lot alike when people would make statements about some of her sensory issues or behaviors. I would point out that she just doesn't mask them as I do and that I envied her for that. Sometimes, this would open up further dialogue about sensory issues in others, and once I got going, I found myself info-dumping. Though not everyone was as excited as I was for these subjects, sometimes I did not care.

I completed various trainings and certifications on autism, although I eventually moved away from them the more I noted ableism in certain aspects. Some were utterly blatant in their attempts to teach masking. I remember one was so rooted in ableism that the majority of it was Applied Behavioral Analysis (ABA) training for Registered Behavior Technicians (RBTs), and this was supposed to be the "Advanced" certification. My disdain for ABA only grew with that, and I messaged the certification commission about the horrendous training and how it was not whatsoever neurodiversity-affirming. I eagerly let that certification lapse. Had I not paid prior to the training, I would not have even completed it. But knowledge still comes with seeing the bad, even if it is knowing what not to do. Any therapy that teaches a child or individual to mask is not a therapy I would allow for my daughter, and it is far from neurodiversity-affirming.

I eventually got involved with autistic-led professional organizations and groups that consisted of many different neurodivergent individuals, many of whom were autistic. I even found other neurodivergent therapists and psychologists in these groups. I started to realize that the concept of being an autistic therapist is really not that far-fetched, and, in some ways, our abilities to identify and read behavioral patterns in others can make us really good therapists. Not to mention, the tendency of autistics to have high somatic or autonomic responsive empathy can also help us during sessions. My own ability to read people has always been advanced. Sometimes, this is simply identifying incongruences in one's verbal and non-verbal behaviors. This is very useful as a therapist.

It was within these groups, as well as many other autistic-led social media groups that I noticed a large number of high-masking individuals, most of whom were late diagnosed. It was also noted in these spaces that these masking behaviors inevitably led to many issues, including shutdown, and while they may have been adapted as a means to blend in, there was a high cost to maintaining or using a mask. Acknowledging one has a mask is the easiest part, but trying to unlearn it is far more difficult. It requires a great deal of mindfulness and awareness of when you use it.

When Devon Price's, *Unmasking Autism: Discovering the New Faces of Neurodiversity* book was released in 2022, it opened up the conversation about this topic more, and many autistic individuals, including myself, started embracing more of their unique traits and behaviors without shame. It hasn't been easy, and it is still an ongoing process. I find that I still put on a mask in various settings, but if I am able to bring up the topic of my autism, then I find I can start being more true to myself. I would highly recommend that book to any other high-maskers like myself.

CHAPTER FIVE

PATHOLOGICAL DEMAND AVOIDANCE

I came across knowledge of pathological demand avoidance (PDA) several years ago when I first started delving into autism. Prior to this, I had never heard of this notion, even as a therapist. Unfortunately, most of the information at that time on PDA was from the United Kingdom, and there was not much knowledge about it here in the United States. Even presently, there is still not a great presence in the US on this topic, and most of those who are prominent advocating voices are found in the UK and Australia. While it is not an official diagnosis, it is considered a subtype or profile of autism that includes individuals who have a significant internal response to the expectations of others or when demands are placed on them. Sadly, this profile has not been universally accepted. More benign terminology such as "demand avoidant" is instead often used.

The National Autistic Society discusses the history of PDA beginning in the 1980s. Professor Elizabeth Newson first coined the term to describe the profile of a group of children she had seen for assessment (National Autistic Society, 2020). She later co-authored the first article on this profile detailing the need for PDA syndrome to have a necessary distinction within the pervasive developmental disorders (Newson et al., 2003). It should be noted that all diagnoses of pervasive developmental disorders are now under the umbrella of autism spectrum disorder (ASD) in the recent updates of the DSM. There has fortunately been quite a bit of research done already on PDA. As an autistic therapist who firmly believes that PDA is a real phenomenon that can cause significant issues in one's daily functioning, I also believe more research is needed to get the information out there front and center to other mental health professionals. I know this because I live this, and I will discuss how it affects me personally further in this chapter. I should also point out another reason for more research is that, unfortunately, there is a disparity of providers with any knowledge of this topic.

Another description that is often used to fit this profile using the same acronym is Persistent Drive for Autonomy, which also fits this very well. I honestly don't have a preference for either because both qualify. The PDA Society, also located in the UK, has a lot of great resources and information on this topic. They detail how autistic individuals with this profile will avoid demands or situations that can trigger extreme anxiety or sensory overwhelm, disrupt routines, affect transitions, or events/activities that they might not see the point of or have any interest in by refusing, withdrawing, shutting down, or escaping in order to avoid these situations (PDA Society, 2022).

Pathological demand avoidance is not a one-size-fits-all profile. How it manifests in each individual varies based on the neurology of that particular person. Some presentations are more internalized and passive — where difficulties are masked; externalized presentations, where there are clear behavioral reactions to the demands, such as aggressive and controlling behavior; and variable presentations that are a mix of both and dependent on various triggers such as environment and setting (PDA Society, 2022). Individuals who do not have this presentation are vastly unaware of just how many things in our daily lives are actual demands. However, before I get into the different types of PDA, I want to discuss my own PDA, even if it's just an iceberg version.

MY PDA PROFILE

As a child, I was mostly a passive internalized demand avoider or fawner. I remember how being told by adults to do things caused me anxiety. Certain tones, especially those of my father, caused me extreme anxiety that I couldn't easily get past. If I got into trouble with teachers it was typically for things I was unaware of, and the heavy shame I felt was excessive. I would have an internal dialogue about how to avoid this situation in the future. As a teen, this continued, but I began managing it better by anticipating expectations. I always had chores assigned to me from pretty early on. I didn't wait until I was told to do them before I completed them.

When I began driving, I found that I made sure to arrive very early for everything. I found if I even felt like I was coming close to being late, I would have super high anxiety. This was rather complicated at one point when I had to drive one of my good friends to school daily, and she was the quintessential undiagnosed ADHD procrastinator. I remember arriving at her home most mornings and having to get her out of bed, tell her to get into the shower, and then brush her teeth. We were never late, however. I made sure of it. Ironically, my avoidance of being late pushed me to place demands on my friend. Luckily, I don't believe she struggled with them as I do. But looking back, I am sure there were many times I would project my demand avoidance onto others by unintentionally being demanding.

As an adult, my demand avoidance only increased, presumably as more demands were being placed on me. The NAVY was in demand all the time. I was internally anxious all the time. Trying to avoid it was very difficult because I would get yelled at for the littlest things that I was unaware I was even doing. I honestly believe trying to cope with this internally only amplified my seizures. Even my people-pleasing tendencies were caused by the fear of someone demanding something of me.

In college and in jobs, I found that I attempted to complete tasks early in order to avoid the demands that being late or procrastinating would inevitably cause. This helped me to be very efficient. Still, as life goes, I wasn't able to avoid the feeling of demand completely. If a professor or boss corrected me on something, I felt it. The older I got, though, the more my PDA started to manifest itself externally. In addition to the extreme anxiety I had previously felt, I now felt intense anger during triggering events. I became more brazen to question certain rules as to the reasoning behind them. I challenged expectations if I felt they were impossible to meet, especially since I felt as though I was very thorough and efficient in all things I did. If I struggled to meet the time of a required task, I felt there was something wrong with the system, and I would say something.

This is the primary reason I ended up transitioning from an agency/hospital setting to contract work. The lack of autonomy in the former was immense, and it was amplified by the disgust at those making the rules who were the ones unaware of how it affected client and therapist care and only cared about the bottom dollar. From contract work, I managed to launch my private practice, wherein I got to be my own boss. I find it is only because of this that I am doing as well as I am now.

If you haven't noticed a theme yet with my PDA, I'll break it down for you: I am a demand avoider by attempting to stay ahead of the demand. I am my own boss. I set my own schedule. I try to control a great number of variables before the variables are placed on me by something else entirely. I have somehow fooled myself into believing if I control the narrative, the narrative doesn't control me. Well, I do believe this overcompensation has helped quell a lot of demands placed on me, so it isn't completely for naught. However, it is not foolproof, and it does not help me avoid all demands.

This tendency to try and stay ahead of the demand may also be a form of a fawning response. If I have a lot of emails, voicemails, or tasks that fall on me at the same time, all are seen as demands, and I immediately feel the dysregulation. My mind tells me to address them immediately because I cannot have them waiting on me. As a result, I end up feeling as if I have a bunch of tabs open, and I have to address each and every one before I can close them all out. The dysregulation and anxiety I feel are very intense until all tasks or demands are addressed. Only then will the anxiety go away, but I am then left with the sheer exhaustion that this response can bring. So, while this response is not openly obvious to others, it is clearly a functional issue for me. It may help me be more efficient during the tasks, but the emotional toll it takes is vast.

My husband's tone has probably caused this to manifest the most in my adult life. Unlike I was as a child, I don't sit quietly, internalizing someone's tone toward me. Instead, I will react or respond to it every time. We are past the ignorance of understanding why I have the reaction to his tone, so now when I hear it, I simply say, "Manage your tone," which is code for "You're setting off my PDA and need to stop right now." Most of his tone comes from the projection of frustration at whatever he is dealing with, which is usually not me. I just happened to ask him a question at that time, and he responds tersely, which my brain perceives as a demand.

On the rare occasion, I get pulled over by a cop, my PDA comes out the worst. It is a running joke in my family to not be present should I ever get pulled over. Immediately, my amygdala response kicks into the fight response, which is my go-to amygdala response to any perceived threat. I can control it to a point, but at minimum, it comes out in a tone. But because I am now aware of my PDA, I will immediately start preparing myself internally for this response and then simply apologizing to them in advance by either saying I am not mad at them but mad at myself (or, in some cases, my husband for not putting my updated registration sticker on like he should have). During episodes like this that ignite an intense fight response, I find it doesn't take long for me to start to feel the effects of recovery from an adrenaline rush. It's not long after that I will feel completely drained.

There are much smaller but frequent things in my life that cause this demanding feeling to occur; that took some time for me to recognize what triggered my angry reactions. One is if I get tailed in traffic. Another is if I am in line at a store and someone is waiting for me. I hate the feeling of anyone waiting on me. It's also why I am an overly fast walker and do pretty much everything at a speedy pace. If someone is waiting on me in a way that seems as if I am in their way, or if they have standards that are impossible to meet, this will almost always cause me anger.

Decisions are another common demand for me. More specifically, I struggle with decision paralysis in many things. I typically do not want to be the one to choose where to eat. I can't get a tattoo because I cannot find something that I find to be worthy of forever placement on my skin. My fear is I will grow tired of whatever it is. I don't even have a favorite color. I like most colors and find that most are great at different things. My living room has bold colors throughout, with bright pops of blues, greens, oranges, yellows, and reds. However, sometimes I love calming colors and love rooms with those. No one color will ever be my favorite. Things that require a decision are carefully analyzed and then given time to commit to them. With careful analysis, I find I can make a scrupulous decision, but don't ask me to make one spontaneously.

Spontaneous phone calls are demands on me, but even if I am able to answer them, my anxiety about the unexpected causes me to generally let it go to voicemail, where I can then prepare better for when I call them back. I also am not your typical texter or emailer. If you text or email me, I will respond as soon as possible. This goes back to making people wait. There is also the fear that I will forget, and that is not acceptable. I have been told by some that they appreciate this because, apparently, this is not a common thing. Indeed, I am not the only person who has this tendency. Although, I do envy those who do not have this internalized thought process driving them. That must be freeing.

My somatic empathy can also be a demand trigger. An example of this recently occurred during a family vacation, and this was the first time I was able to verbalize to others and myself what was going on internally. As a family of nine, we ventured into a cute little ice cream place. Six of us ordered ice cream, boba drinks, or tea. The place had one employee in it, and as we entered, so did a lot of others. I immediately started feeling anxious. The employee (possibly the owner) was still taking orders about ten minutes after we arrived and had only been able to make one of our drinks. When a gentleman who ordered long after we did was able to get his ice cream immediately, my husband made a look at me. My brain immediately perceived the demand to be placed on me.

In the past, I would have just kept my thoughts to myself. But this particular time, I didn't keep it to myself. I immediately spoke up to my husband and stated, "I know, I know." I then relayed all my thoughts and emotions. I processed all my anxiety and dysregulation. I mentioned how I felt about there being only one employee, knowing she needed help and also feeling the impatience from everyone else in the shop. This, in the past, would have led to me just seemingly being in a bad mood all of a sudden, but this helped educate my family about my struggle. It also reduced the intensity of what I was feeling. It wasn't long after that we all got our order, and upon leaving, I felt lighter. I was able to regulate back to baseline fairly quickly. This one incident showed that I am still learning about all the ways my brain perceives demand.

TYPES OF DEMAND

I am certain that I am not even remotely close to understanding everything that is a demand for me. It isn't until I have an internal or external reaction that I start trying to process through the lens of demand avoidance. I still have ah-ha moments when I make those connections. There are some clear things that are common demands for individuals with PDA, one of which is time. While we prefer structure and stability in regard to time, it can sometimes be a double-edged sword in that the demand sometimes outweighs the structure of a task.

PDAs don't like to be put on the spot unexpectedly. We do not like being asked questions in the middle of class or similar occurrences. Spontaneity is too demanding. Don't ask us to do something today if there is an option to do it at another time. Even fun plans are not fun if there is no time to absorb them. I generally like to schedule things in advance, and I tell my friends, family, and colleagues this as much as possible. The irony of this is I also get anxious when the date draws closer, but I am still able to manage that anxiety a lot easier than if it was spontaneously dropped on me.

Change itself can also bring about a PDA response. Transitions need buffer times to better prepare. This is one reason that I find the "5 minutes left" rule at the end of play therapy sessions to be especially important for neurodivergent children. Again, they still may react to the initial demand of the 5-minute warning, but by the time you have counted down, they generally are more prepared to transition. My daughter is a classic example of this. If you don't do the 5-minute warning, you will most likely end up in meltdown territory as opposed to some initial whining.

Any change will also come with uncertainty. More specifically, according to recent research, intolerance of uncertainty (IoU), a trait characterized by the overvaluation of predictability that comes with the feeling of being overwhelmed by the unknown or unexpected, has been shown to be a significant factor in PDA (Jenkinson et al., 2020). This is why many, such as myself, will overcompensate in order to avoid demand because the aspect of feeling in control helps to minimize IoU.

As I addressed in my own PDA profile, decisions are a common demand-avoidance task for many. Decision paralysis can cause a great deal of struggle with one's daily functioning. Not everyone is able to make a big decision, even with ample time to carefully analyze it. For those with severe forms of this, it is truly paralyzing, and they need to bring in others to help them make these big decisions. Guilting someone for not making a decision only adds another demand to their plate, so please avoid doing that.

The sheer number of demands in this life is daunting. There is no way I could cover them all. That task itself seems too demanding. There are even smaller demands hidden within larger demands. We cannot avoid them all because they are everywhere. Many of these are often unspoken until an autistic individual gets into trouble for not meeting them. Even non-PDAs struggle at times with demands. Some people get annoyed when they have to stop doing something fun in order to eat or go to the restroom; however, for those with PDA, these instances are quite frequent and go beyond the typical annoyed response.

PDA and the Amygdala

Many neurodiversity-affirming therapists believe that Oppositional Defiant Disorder (ODD) is actually PDA. I will admit I really do not like the ODD diagnosis. To me, it is a catch-all term given to any child or teen who doesn't fall within societal norms of accepting authority. It is not trauma-informed, and it is most definitely not neurodivergent-informed. It does not give the why of behavior; rather, it is strictly a label that often attaches an incorrect stigma to the individual prior to even meeting them.

There are also neuroimaging studies that have been done to indicate that the areas of the brain affected during a PDA response are typically the same areas affected during meltdowns. These are also the areas in the brain that trauma can affect. So, while I will not go so far as to say that ODD is probably PDA, I firmly believe that it is either PDA or a PTSD/trauma response. More research is definitely needed on this subject.

Because PDA has not yet been researched as much as we would prefer it to be, we are still lacking a lot of the specific science behind what is going on in the brain and the nervous system of a PDA individual. However, there is enough research to indicate that what is happening in the brain is igniting the fight, flight, freeze, or fawn response. I am not alone when I say that in the PDA brain, the amygdala recognizes "demand" as a genuine threat (Wilding, 2022).

Many mental health professionals, especially play therapists, often call this an amygdala hijack or an amygdala flip. It occurs in the part of the brain that reacts to stress, anger, aggression, or fear by releasing the stress hormones, cortisol and adrenaline, that prepare our body to fight, flight, freeze, or fawn. It does this by sending a distress signal to the hypothalamus, which communicates with the body's autonomic nervous system and its two components, the sympathetic and parasympathetic nervous systems (Harvard Health, 2020).

Many PDA brains react by not complying with a demand. This is the freeze response. It is not a choice when an individual reacts this way. This is the most common reaction to PDA that I see in my clients. The flight reaction typically follows this when the individual tries to evade the task altogether. The fawn response occurs when the individual tries to please people, and it may be more difficult to notice because the behavior is typically what the demander desires. It's only the feelings and emotions that the PDA individual feels internally that would alert them to this being a stress response. This includes feeling not only the stress hormones but also possibly nausea or extreme exhaustion up to hours or days later.

This delayed reaction can cause significant confusion for family members, friends, colleagues, or support of the autistic individual.

I feel this was my early childhood reaction to demand. However, as an adult, it has flipped to mostly the fight response, which comes out in anger. Even during my fawning approach to staying ahead of the demand, my dysregulation often included feelings of anger. While I control it to the best of my capability, the internal anger response definitely feels like a hijacking experience. My tone is not very controlled, and ideally, I try to avoid talking to anyone at that time if I can help it. Unfortunately, that is not always a possibility, such as when I get pulled over by a cop. I honestly just wish I had the nervous system response many non-PDAs or non-traumatized individuals have. I have no doubt that if I would have had this type of response as a child, I would have been given an ODD diagnosis.

Knowing what is going on inside the brain and body of a child with PDA is very important in helping to support them. Traditional approaches and discipline are the exact opposite of what these children need. If you see their behavior as simply the result of an amygdala hijack and nervous system response, you can see how those approaches would actually lead to increased adverse behaviors in the child.

There have been occasions where I have received a stressful, aggressive email that has ignited this demand response. This is why I prefer email as a primary mode of communication because I can then take several moments to calm down before I respond. But even when I do finally sit down, even if it is the next day to write a response, I find the amygdala reactions still occur, however, they are less intense. I still feel the adrenaline pumping through me, and I have to ask my husband or another close party to see if my response is composed enough. Sometimes it is, but other times they will tell me to tone it down. Even with written expression being my ideal mode of communication, this amygdala response can cause me to be more emotional and less logical during these times.

There are several great bloggers, professionals, and PDA activists that openly share their struggle with PDA in hopes to try and get the word out (see the "Resources" section for examples). There are quite a few voices out there, and one can learn a great deal from their stories. Individuals with PDA, often called PDAs, can struggle quite frequently with meltdowns and shutdowns. In my own experience, demands have been the cause of my biggest meltdowns which have consequently led to my most intense acute shutdowns.

Some of my clients have also processed this to be the case for them. Several have sought me out specifically because of my knowledge and lived experience of this issue. Ideally, we need more therapists and other professionals aware of this as well, especially in educational, medical, and therapeutic settings. While it is not a formal diagnosis, it can detail a specific struggle and profile of individuals that have it affect their daily functioning.

Chapter Six

Trauma

The subject of trauma should be included in all books related to autism. And yes, when I talk about autistic shutdown, there will most definitely be a whole chapter devoted to this complex trigger, even if it is just an iceberg of the topic. Trauma changes brains and autistic brains are more at risk for trauma and its effects because of various complexities that I will be discussing throughout this chapter. There is not a mental health professional out there who hasn't worked with trauma in some form. Some therapists will specialize in this and have done a vast amount of training to be able to treat the different types of trauma.

Unfortunately, I have noticed that there are not enough therapists or mental health professionals with specific training in trauma and autistic brain, particularly utilizing a neurodiversity-affirming perspective. This is partly because it is hard to find such training. I have had to really dig to find training online that meets this need in the past, and I don't even remember the last time one was offered in my state. Interestingly enough, there is actually quite a bit of research out there on this topic, but it just hasn't been put in the right hands because of the lack of training opportunities. Sadly, many wrongfully believe because they don't "work with" this population that it isn't needed. But, part of such training discusses how some individuals have been misdiagnosed because of some of the overlapping symptoms of autism and Post-Traumatic Stress Disorder (PTSD). In some cases, individuals can even have both. One research on this topic showed probable PTSD in autistics to range from 43% to 45% (Rumball, 2020).

Let's review a typical scenario of what happens when any child enters therapy for problematic behaviors with no previous diagnosis: During the intake, the mental health professional will review a number of questions, inevitably leading up to the question about traumas. The parent or caregiver will detail some very specific major traumas, which can include abandonment as an infant, abuse or neglect, witnessing a traumatic incident, being severely injured, loss of a parent or sibling, etc. You get the idea that any number of traumatic things can occur to a child at a young age.

Once the trauma is detailed to the therapist, they immediately begin breaking down how they believe that relates to their behaviors. They're reviewing attachment theory and breaking down what therapeutic interventions may be needed depending on their age and a number of other factors. Some will go in more depth, asking about possible head injuries, which is definitely important. But, along the way, no questions are ever asked about sensory struggles, social or communication issues, or maybe repetitive behaviors or tics.

Let's look at this same scenario but with a teen or adult: There's no real difference, with the exceptions being that the presenting issue might be depression or another mental health struggle, and it is not the parents being asked the questions but the clients themselves. The same thought process is going through the therapist's mind, even down to attachment theory for some. But again, there are no questions that might highlight the possibility that an autism diagnosis might be underlying. Why is this important? Without knowing or understanding that an individual might have an autistic brain, a therapist will miss a significant aspect of treatment, including the knowledge of autistic shutdown. This is particularly important if trauma is involved, but also it is important to note autistic brains will perceive some things to be traumas that are not typical with allistics.

INCREASED RISK

There is an increased risk for autistic individuals to be exposed to traumatic life events, particularly interpersonal traumas such as physical and sexual abuse, and bullying (Rumball, 2022). Bullying is a difficult one because it happens so frequently, and many children and teens choose not to be forthcoming to their caretakers or, due to their limited verbal ability, may be unable to inform them of an incident. Some studies have shown that up to 70 percent of autistic children who are mainstreamed are bullied, and 46% of autistic kids in middle and high school have reported being victimized (Verret,

2016). By the time bullying is identified, a significant amount of trauma has been endured.

Bullying of various types can also occur as an adult in diverse settings such as college and places of employment. Alienation of these individuals or lack of support often adds to the increase in exposure to interpersonal traumas in general population settings (Brewin et al., 2000). Other examples of social, communication, and other interpersonal issues include extreme social difficulties and confusion from individuals misinterpreting social cues that may lead to an increased tendency to be misunderstood, therefore increasing the likelihood of conflict to occur (Rumball, 2022). Even the aspect of conflict arising in a simple situation can lead to a traumatic experience for autistic individuals.

The other two specific issues that should be included in every intake are sensory struggles and repetitive behaviors or tics. Each one of these, regardless of a formal diagnosis, are characteristics that are more likely to expose an individual to traumatic experiences. The sensory processing system of an autistic individual or someone who has Sensory Processing Disorder (SPD) works differently than that of allistic individuals. Emma from Undercover Autism (2020) gives an excellent description of what sensory trauma feels like. They describe that even the way they perceive the world through their senses is traumatic because the repeated exposure to daily unavoidable pain makes their body react as if it is in danger from a threat (Emma, 2020). My own sensory sensitivities have shown this to be true in my case as well.

Repetitious behaviors such as stims can be alienating at times, but just the aspect of trying to suppress or restrict an individual's stims can be traumatic over time. Tics are involuntary, however, and therefore are not included in that because one cannot mask them. The opposite issue tends to occur with individuals who have tics. Their trauma occurs from the physical and emotional toil that tics can put on the individual who has them. Unfortunately, research has proven this as individuals with Tourette's and chronic tic disorders are associated with having a substantial risk of suicide (Fernández de la Cruz et al., 2017).

There is also the aspect of how some of the autistic everyday struggles can lead to real internal trauma responses, such as what was previously described regarding transitions, meltdowns, and demands. It is also imperative to note the concern for racial and intergenerational trauma as both have daily systemic complexities that are rampant throughout our cultures and place autistic Black, Indigenous, and people of color (BIPOC) at even higher risk for trauma. The brain is definitely being affected in all of these situations. Shutdowns often occur as an acute response to these traumas. Therapy can be a great resource for processing when such incidents occur because, over time, they will increase the chances of complex PTSD (C-PTSD) if untreated.

RELIGIOUS TRAUMA

Over the past several years, I personally have seen an uptick in the number of individuals struggling with religious trauma. I understand where they are coming from, even as a non-denominational follower of Jesus who grew up in church. Autistics and other neurodivergent individuals are especially vulnerable to this abuse. I personally do not really consider myself religious, but I am definitely more on the spiritual side of things. Religion in itself often rubs me the wrong way, especially when it is weaponized. However, I do believe in Jesus and his teachings of love.

One aspect of religious trauma includes the increased likelihood that autistic individuals will identify as LGBTQIA+ and many religions have made it their point to disparage these individuals. Research has shown autistic adults and adolescents are approximately eight times more likely to identify as asexual and 'other' sexes than their non-autistic peers (Weir et al., 2021). Imagine that! The same brain that these individuals are born with that makes them autistic is the same brain that makes them up to 80% more likely than allistics to identify as something other than heterosexual.

Inevitably, when these individuals come out with their identities to their religious families and friends, they are often told they are going to hell, and many others are disowned and discarded as if they committed the worst atrocities imaginable, all because of who they want to be or who they want to be with. Many are being treated this way by so-called Christians and other religions that see nothing wrong with the hate they dispense, their own judging behaviors, and the multitude of "sins" that they commit on a daily basis. Some of these include process addictions, substance use issues, adultery, mistreatment of their own spouses, and especially the treatment of women in general. It seems the "love thy neighbor" part of the Bible gets forsaken by these individuals.

This seems like an excellent time to discuss the tendency for many autistic individuals to have a high justice principle. Research has even shown that autistics have an altered pattern of moral behavior, which is closely associated with functional changes in the right temporoparietal junction (rTPJ), leading these individuals to be more inflexible when following a moral rule, even if the immoral action would benefit themselves because of increased concern about their ill-gotten gains and moral cost (Hu et al., 2020). In essence, they are more likely to do what they feel is the right thing, even at their own expense.

NeuroClastic (2020) gave an interesting perspective that autistic people were more likely to be selfless and show more integrity in their moral values than neurotypical people and were less likely to change their moral values based on their own individual gain, even if that gain was large, and they generally care more about their own values than themselves, which is seemingly the opposite of neurotypical people. I personally have noted many autistics make some of the best advocates because of this tendency. They are used to standing alone and being alienated at times, but they still continue to stand. Many of these individuals are also part of other minority groups that have been treated as unequal, such as those who are BIPOC or are simply women. These individuals will speak up on the inequality that they see in whatever setting they see it in.

I discussed in an earlier section of this book about autistics, noting incongruences in behaviors. Many autistic individuals have noted a compelling incongruence in the behaviors of these religious individuals who dictate judgment towards LGBTQIA+ and other minority groups and the religion they claim to be dictating from. In short, they are noting hypocrisy, and this hypocrisy is turning them away. It saddens me that for many who make their way to my office, I may be the one person of faith in their life who affirms their brain and their individuality. On the rare occasion, I have a friend or family member who asks me about this, I firmly state that I have seen more individuals turn away from God because of their treatment by these so-called Christians, and if they think that is acceptable, then they are not the followers of Jesus they think they are.

Other facets of religious trauma include the number of demands that many religions have. Combine that with an individual already predisposed to have a trauma response such as PDA, and you have a detrimental mix. Heavy shame is also the focus of many religions. This can be especially hard on individuals who already have heavy shame meters, such as many autistics. According to research on shame, it is at the core of the symptomatology of Post-Traumatic Stress Disorder (Arel, 2018).

The perplexity of shame in religion is that it is often disguised or attributed to being necessary because it is based on love. According to further research, family and religious community dynamics may be structured by chronic shame, even when the individual in the community feels love, and religious shaming, particularly Christian shaming, is routinely and consistently presented and justified as love (Downie, 2022). A statement from parents that is a prime example of this is, "I am doing this because I love you." Many autistics who tend to be concrete thinkers have difficulty making sense of such statements as these and find the incongruence of the statements to be hypocritical as they grow older.

Autistics are obviously not the only individuals to have religious trauma, and the issue goes much deeper than the few paragraphs I can give in this book. This issue continues to grow in magnitude, and whether it's because of politics or social media does not matter. What matters is it is happening, and it is causing real pain and turmoil in these individuals' lives and their mental health. Many of these individuals have felt marginalized, been guilted for not attending church or choosing to leave altogether, and in simply unfathomable situations have been physically or sexually abused by religious leaders or those protected by religious leaders. There are of course many other ways that religious trauma can occur including being a part of or leaving cults. It is important for us to recognize this as a significant problem and one that can most definitely lead to C-PTSD.

Trauma Treatments

Eye Movement Desensitization and Reprocessing (EMDR)

There are some great therapeutic modalities that have had great success with autistic trauma, along with talk therapy for those who desire it. One that I have been trained in and employ frequently is Eye Movement Desensitization and Reprocessing (EMDR). EMDR has become an ideal treatment for PTSD symptoms and other disturbing life experiences. It was created by Francine Shapiro in 1987 after a walk. During the walk, she noticed that as she moved her eyes back and forth, the negative thoughts that she had been having were decreasing.

As she began looking into it further, she noted that it wasn't just the aspect of the eye movements that worked alone. It was only in combination with certain cognitive components that the negative thoughts would decrease. She created the original standard procedure, Eye Movement Desensitization (EMD), soon after. She continued to develop an 8-stage protocol, which we now know as EMDR, in 1991 after incorporating feedback from clients and other therapists. Numerous research and case studies have been concluded since the original EMD protocol was designed. Further research and numerous outcome studies since the EMDR approach was created, have shown that in comparison to talk psychotherapy, EMDR therapy can produce effective results much more quickly.

According to the EMDR website, EMDR therapy can help the mind heal from psychological trauma, similar to how the body can recover from physical trauma by removing blocks that are impeding the healing (2020). I am a metaphor person, and some individuals often struggle with the science behind it, so I use the metaphor of a tree with a frisbee caught in a limb. The frisbee is like a trauma; only it is preventing the limbs from doing their job: holding up all the leaves and squirrels. EMDR is a way to shake up those limbs using bilateral stimulation. That bilateral stimulation is guided by the therapist and can come in the form of eye movement, tactile (using hand devices such as buzzers), or self-tapping, or auditory using sounds through headphones.

My preference is using hand tappers or buzzers because I like the aspect that the individual can close their eyes. However, I give the client the option to choose a different stimulation modality if they find that the tappers mess with their sensory issues. My second most popular stimulation modality is guided self-tapping, which can also be used through telehealth. The least used is the two-finger hand to guide their eyes back and forth.

EMDR is an ideal trauma modality for individuals who struggle with talk therapy because it doesn't necessarily require the individual to detail the event or trauma to the therapist. This is fitting for those with pragmatic communication disorders or even those such as veterans who can't or won't disclose the exact nature of the trauma. I can find workarounds for Stage 1 (History and Treatment Planning), Stage 3 (Assessment), and Stage 4 (Desensitization) if the verbal aspect is an impediment.

EMDR doesn't take the memory away. The goal is to decrease the emotional disturbance, autonomic and visceral nervous reactions attached to the memory. It can also be used in things that some individuals may not consider trauma but still may be disturbing to them. And yes, it can help even C-PTSD. With autistic individuals, it can also be used to help with social interactions and high anxiety caused by certain triggers. I have included some great EMDR resources and video links in the resources section towards the end of this book. One of the videos is that of an autistic individual's experience and their description of the therapeutic modality, which they break down very well.

One unfortunate aspect of EMDR is that it is not consistently available in all areas, as limited therapists in some states are actually trained in it. In our state, particularly the region I live in, there are many who are trained, but in Oklahoma, where I am from, I have been unable to locate one needed for close family and friends. One of the only other downsides to this treatment modality is actually one of its benefits. As therapy progresses, it is not uncommon for repressed past traumas to resurface. This is not done deliberately. Our brains are amazing things, and often, repression is done as a form of protection when it knows we may not have the capability of managing the severity of trauma at this point in time. So, it might lock it away for a bit.

As our brains start to heal with EMDR, we work with a particular memory or trauma that might unlock another. This trauma might be related, or it might just be the brain healing and thus allowing another trauma to be addressed. If this happens in a session, a therapist will guide the client to use the appropriate resource, such as a container, to put it away until the next session when it can be addressed. Resourcing is typically done before EMDR sessions begin. I typically review up to three resources that a client can draw upon either during the session or anytime outside of sessions as a general coping skill. My three favorites are container, safe place, and nurturing figure, but there are others as well.

My thoughts on EMDR include my hope that it will one day be readily available in all states and regions. I feel that it should be a prominent treatment in all veteran hospitals and clinics. I would love to see it be a prescribed treatment given by Doctors and hospitals to individuals who are struggling with things from accidents, illness, sick family members, and chronic pain issues, much like they prescribe medication or physical therapy. I wholeheartedly believe that things such as Chronic Regional Pain Syndrome (CRPS) would be mitigated or prevented in many cases, as well as PTSD.

Neurofeedback

Neurofeedback is a treatment modality that I haven't been trained in yet, but it is something I am interested in. Neurofeedback, also known as Neurotherapy, is a modality that helps clients control their brain waves consciously using electroencephalogram (EEG) biofeedback to help treat things such as depression, anxiety, PTSD, addiction, focus issues, and self-regulation. It has also been known to help treat brain damage from brain injuries such as tumors and strokes and movement disorders such as Parkinson's disease. Using a computer-based system to map brain waves and non-invasively record electrical activity on the scalp as it is paired with visual and audio signals, such as a computer game, in an effort to try and retrain the brain (Cunha, 2022).

It does sound a bit complex, but also very promising. Unfortunately, it is not a common modality—even less common than EMDR—and it can be rather difficult to find a therapist who is trained in it. Another downside is that it can be time-consuming and, unlike EMDR, can take months to achieve results, and results are not permanent (Cunha, 2022).

It is a much older therapy than EMDR, with its roots going all the way back to the 1950s and '60s by Dr. Joe Kamiya and Dr. Barry Sterman. According to Brainworks (2022), around the same time Dr. Kamiya was studying consciousness and learning simple reward systems could help people learn to alter their brain activity, Dr. Sterman was running an experiment on cats to see if there could be an increase in their sensory-motor rhythm (SMR) by providing food pellets for correct responses and inevitably leading to the cats learning to control their brainwaves to get the treat.

According to Myndlift's (2022) research, he further expanded when he was performing an experiment for NASA on whether rocket fuel caused seizures. He used some of the same cats from his previous research and discovered that those cats were significantly less likely to experience seizures than other cats who did not undergo SMR training. This led to further research outcomes on humans, indicating that 60% of the subjects were able to reduce their epileptic seizures by 20-100%, which was long-lasting (Myndlift, 2022). As someone who has undergone horrible medication therapy for epilepsy, I find the notion of a treatment like this very auspicious. I am curious why it isn't a go-to therapy prescribed by doctors, considering some medications are harmful to one's liver, such as the one that I took.

Controlled studies on children and adolescents began in the '70s for the treatment of ADHD and further expanded in the '80s. It was in the '90s that brought about treatments for other psychological disorders and central nervous system-based conditions (Brainworks, 2022). Much of the neuroscience behind neurofeedback falls under the theory of neuroplasticity. This is the ability of the nervous system to change its activity in response to intrinsic or extrinsic stimuli by reorganizing its functions, structure, or connections, which can occur at any age (Mateos-Aparicio & Rodríguez-Moreno, 2019).

The concept of whether or not new neurons can form in adulthood has been something that has been debated in the scientific community. Some of the most recent research. However, has indicated that neurogenesis is possible in the area of the brain that is responsible for memory, mood regulation, and learning (Weintraub, 2019). While there are still those who have doubts, I would surmise that Neurofeedback has shown that it is highly likely that neurogenesis is occurring in adult brains.

Neurofeedback video descriptions are readily available on YouTube. I have included my favorite in the resources section of this book. Even considering the downsides to this therapy, I feel there are a lot of advantages to it. I personally find it tempting to find a practitioner for myself.

There are, of course, other therapies that can be beneficial in treating trauma. I chose to highlight these two, considering their application to autistic individuals' brains and how they might be more favorable for those who might have limitations in pragmatic or verbal speech. I would also fall into that category at times. Like my own needs, I have some clients that vacillate between talk therapy and EMDR simply because some days they aren't able to articulate themselves well, and this option is great for that.

Remember that autism is a dynamic disability, and our functioning ability fluctuates. We need modalities that can be adjusted as needed. There are a great many talk therapy theories, treatments, and modalities that can be beneficial for treating trauma. I do not align with just one as every individual is unique and requires an approach catered to their specific needs. If you find yourself with a therapist who pushes a specific modality that doesn't align with your needs, feel free to speak up. Many will adjust, but if they do not, please do not hesitate to keep looking for one that is a better fit for you.

Trauma and Shutdown

Unfortunately, there is no shortage of traumas in this life. And everyone has dealt with some form or other of trauma. In mental health, we often distinguish traumas as either "little T" or "big T" traumas. The latter are those that are considered major traumas such as those sexual in nature or being a witness to a crime. The former are those that might seem more minor in comparison, such as being in a fender bender or getting fired from a job. Both can be damaging and leave significant scars. And what one individual can cope with is not what another individual can necessarily endure.

The autistic brain adds various complexities of not only how it handles traumas but what may constitute trauma for an autistic individual. Sometimes an autistic individual may not even realize how damaging a situation was until later when they are in meltdown or shutdown. It's only in hindsight that they might consider what they weathered as a trauma. Considering the PFC takes a rather large hit during trauma, it's no big revelation that an autistic individual will be at risk for increased meltdowns and shutdowns.

Chapter Seven

OTHER SPECIAL CONSIDERATIONS AND POPULATIONS

While the object of this book is to detail the experience of the autistic shutdown, I definitely wanted to highlight several different populations and prominent subject areas that I feel are particularly crucial to note. Many of these have been brought to my attention by various clients of mine and their own lived experiences. It is quite possible, even if you do not think any of these topics are relevant to you, that you might note something that corresponds to some of your own lived experiences. Even if it doesn't relate to you specifically, autistic individuals around you could likely use this information in some way.

WOMEN

In my practice, I have observed the highest number of late-diagnosed adults to be more likely assigned female at birth (AFAB) or transgender women. The diagnosis ratio of males to females diagnosed with autism has generally been 4:1. However, there is a proportion of professionals who are starting to believe that the number is more likely to be equal, considering the high percentage of high masking females that are not being diagnosed until later in life. Considering what I have seen in my own practice, I also believe this to be highly plausible.

I have also noted that the people that I have worked with the most on autistic shutdown happen to be women. I have two thoughts on the reasoning behind this:

1. Women are more likely to reach out for therapy in general. So yes, relatively speaking, I am more likely going to see women dealing with shutdown.

2. There are unique complexities as women that make us more likely to struggle with shutdowns.

And those complexities are what I will be addressing.

Hormonal Aspect

As noted in the first part of this book, I mentioned my own issues related to how menstruation can often add complications to an autistic individual's lived experience. These factors have not decreased as I have aged but have increased over the years, leading to a uterine ablation several years ago that has given me much of my life back. Before that, I had to work my whole life around that time of the month, and it was definitely affecting my daily functioning during that time. Even my issues with progesterone that caused multiple miscarriages and devastating losses can be attributed to my already faulty hormonal system.

Research has begun to identify a correlation between autistic women having an increase in hormonal-related issues. Some of these issues include Premenstrual dysphoric disorder (PMDD) and Polycystic ovary syndrome (PCOS), which are two of the most common issues I have seen with my own clientele. There is also an increased likelihood for autistic women to experience an increase in menopause symptoms and overall menopause complaints, including psychological complaints such as anxiety, depression, inattention, impulsivity, and other autistic characteristics (Groenman et al., 2021).

Premenstrual dysphoric disorder (PMDD) occurs in the week leading up to menstruation, which is also the week that premenstrual syndrome (PMS) typically occurs. Even in typical individuals, symptoms that can occur during this time include irritability, low mood and energy, and painful breasts. Five to eight percent of women who menstruate, however, will experience emotional and physical symptoms that are more debilitating and affect their daily functioning due to PMDD (Groenman, 2022). Various research has indicated that autistic individuals have an increased risk of PMDD, with disparate prevalence rates depending on the research. One particular study suggests the prevalence of PMDD to be 92% in the autism group compared with 11% in the control group (Obaydi & Puri, 2008). Others showed significance, though not as drastic.

Personally, I have a few clients in my own practice who have PMDD and are either diagnosed officially or are self-diagnosed autistic. I have had one client who has stated this to be their biggest struggle as an autistic/ADHD individual. They report the hardest times to cope and the highest likelihood of shutdowns happening during this week every month and have even contemplated permanent solutions to avoid this entirely. Considering the intensity of their symptoms, it is no wonder why they would consider that. PMDD is very debilitating.

Polycystic ovary syndrome (PCOS) is another hormonal disorder marked by an increase in the number of androgens (male sex hormones), causing the individual to have cysts form inside the ovaries. This can cause symptoms ranging from insulin resistance, weight gain, missed/irregular periods, excess body hair, infertility, acne, thinning hair, etc. Two studies found an increased prevalence of PCOS in autistic women, as well as a third study, found significantly increased odds of women with PCOS having an autistic child, even after adjustment for maternal psychiatric diagnoses, obstetric complications, and maternal metabolic conditions (Nover, 2022).

Many of the articles that discussed the correlation between women with PCOS and having autistic children suggested that this link was due to the increase in testosterone in these women; however, none of these studies even considered the possibility that the mother with PCOS was potentially an undiagnosed autistic as well, which would also explain the high hereditary component overall. Even the Center for Disease Control (CDC) has stated that if someone in one's family is autistic, that one may be more likely to have an autistic child (2022). This is a classic example of correlation doesn't always equal causation—so many of these researchers are too busy trying to find a medical cause for these children being autistic that they missed the possibility of the mothers themselves being autistic. Either way, I have personally noted several autistic women in my practice and in online autistic groups who have struggled with PCOS as well as other hormonal issues.

Other research has consistently found autistic women to be more at risk of a variety of different hormonal and medical diagnoses. The results of one study did suggest a link between autistic women having an increased risk of medical conditions and physical symptoms that relate to sex-steroid functions such as reproductive system diagnoses, prediabetes symptoms, earlier puberty onset, PCOS, PMS, and menstrual irregularities, as well as a significant risk of having anovulation, ovarian cancer, and uterine cancer (Simantov et al., 2021). When we consider the consequences for many of these issues, it's no wonder at all how it might be evident that they would affect one's mood, behavior, and daily functioning. Addressing the hormonal aspect should, therefore, be a conventional method of treatment for autistic women. Luckily, it looks like there are some doctors that are making efforts to do this.

Doctors from Richmond Behavioral Associates, NY, are actively researching the possibility of autistic women having an imbalance in two hormones, oxytocin and vasopressin, that might be leading to some issues associated with sensory processing and social bonding (Datta, 2017). The ultimate goal of the Datta research is to improve the quality of life for these women utilizing a nasal spray hormonal medication, which has been shown to improve auditory recall, learning senses, and sensory overload and thus far has shown no adverse effects. While this is only one study of hormonal treatment that could be beneficial to improve the quality of life of some, there is definitely hope that more will also come about to address the other various hormonal struggles of autistic women that affect us on a daily basis.

Parenting (Men included)

Looking back at my childhood and teen years, there were definite signs and struggles I possessed that indicated the likelihood of being autistic. However, it wasn't until I became a mother that many of my most significant symptoms started to manifest on a more regular basis. More significant is the fact that I was less likely to mask. While I did not struggle with Postpartum depression (PPD), I definitely had a lot of Postpartum anxiety (PPA), which hit the first night I brought my oldest home from the hospital. I found I was unable to sleep at all until I found a way to safely co-sleep. Crying wasn't something that I was able to sit through.

Even as a very young mother at 20, I found I aligned with attachment style parenting, not even knowing at the time that's what it was. However, I found that I was able to quell baby cries by meeting their needs fairly quickly. If I didn't know what their need was, I went into detective mode and eventually figured it out. Only one of my children had an aspect of colic, and that was my youngest. Every night around 6:00, she would start a crying spell where I would hold her close and bounce with her on a yoga ball for hours, which curbed the crying so long as I was bouncing. However, I needed to get to the root of what was going on. I wasn't going to just assume that some children get colic. There was a cause, and I was going to figure it out. I didn't see any indication of tummy troubles, but I figured if something was coming from my breast milk, I needed to figure out what it was. So, I went on an elimination diet and removed the first thing I could think of: my morning coffee. The very next day, she didn't cry. So, I switched to decaf, and from there on out, she never had another bout of crying.

I realize now that even though it took hours to get into her system, one cup of coffee was too much for her nervous system. None of my other children ever had any issues with it, but this one did, and I did not drink caffeine for a full year. I did not wean her after a year, but she ate enough solid foods that I figured she might not have the issues, and I was correct. I obsessed over that entire year, though. Obsession, in general, occurred the most after I became a parent, particularly with anything that involved being a parent. It is one of the reasons I nursed my children for so long in general. It is also why I was not able to leave them with someone else for very long at all. My fears spread to a number of things.

Sensory overwhelm also hit hard after having my first. While it was more the crying than anything, I found I was mapping out my travels to limit exposure to crowds. While avoiding illness was one reason behind that, the primary motive was to avoid noise and people. Walmart's weren't especially awful in Oklahoma, but the same was not true when we moved to Arkansas, and it has only gotten worse over the years because of the growth in this area. Taking them to places to play was limited based on whether the park or wherever else was busy.

I remember trying to plan some playdates because I felt some loneliness at times, but when the event came up, I would struggle with social anxiety and would inevitably just stop doing them. Looking back, I think things would have definitely been different for me if I had known I was autistic. For one, I wouldn't have even tried to force myself to do these things that were often considered normal parenting things, such as play dates.

Transitions were another big undertaking. I am a very logistic-minded individual, and I never like to do anything without decent planning. But as a parent of a baby, planning was even more overwhelming. It required packing a huge number of things for the simplest of tasks. I found I was unable to put more than two errands on my plate a day if it involved bringing a baby. At home, I found that I was switching from task to task too quickly for my own comfort because of the needs of the baby, and that would cause me high anxiety due in part to my demand avoidance. I still struggle with this, but I at least have gotten somewhat more comfortable with it over the last 22 years of being a parent. I still prefer planned transitions, though.

My experience as an autistic mother is not that uncommon. Many autistic women report that many of their symptoms got worse when they became a mother. It is a fairly common trigger to shutdowns that I have noticed within my own practice, and especially for myself, it is a big one.

According to research, autistic mothers are more likely to experience additional psychiatric conditions such as pre- or post-partum depression, report greater difficulties in areas such as multitasking, coping with domestic responsibilities, and creating social opportunities for their child, and are more likely to have higher rates of selective mutism, higher anxiety, and find motherhood isolating (Pohl et al., 2020). I honestly believe more grace for ourselves as mothers can go a long way in general, but as autistic women, we need this grace more than anyone. Don't hesitate at all to reach out for support if you are struggling. Friends, family, parenting, and autism groups are all a means of support. Even if it is online, it can often be a big help.

I should also point out that the parenting dilemma is not just a women's issue. Men can definitely deal with a decrease in their overall functioning from parenting, and it can lead to a shutdown, just as well. The hormonal aspect of things amplifies it in women. It is also more common for women to be the primary caretakers. However, this is beginning to decrease in our culture. In fact, due to many women out-earning their male partners in 2021, 2.1 million fathers were stay-at-home dads, up 8% since 1989, according to the Pew Research Center (Kelly, 2022), so this section can also apply to men.

COMMON COMORBIDITIES OR OTHER DISABILITIES

It is rare for autism to be a stand-alone condition in most individuals. Even if nothing else is officially diagnosed, there is a high chance that an individual has another disorder that can be found in the DSM, other medical diagnoses, or both. I have already mentioned several other common comorbidities that autistic individuals might have in addition. Every comorbidity an autistic individual has adds complexities to their daily life and overall ability to function. Some of them affect the individual a great deal and can add a layer of frustration to an already taxed system. These individuals have to take additional care of themselves to prevent things like shutdown, as many of these conditions make them predisposed to shutting down more easily than neurotypical individuals. There is no way I could fit all of these in this book, but I will highlight a few of those that are among the most common.

Attention Deficit Hyperactivity Disorder (ADHD) is one of the most common ones and accounts for 30%-50% of autistic people (Matusiak, 2020). While there is an overlap in symptoms between the two, individuals can definitely have both. My daughter, who is autistic, received her ADHD diagnosis at the age of 9. My preference would be to have all individuals who are being tested for autism also have ADHD testing included and vice versa. I say this because many individuals who get tested for one only realize later that some of their issues are actually from the other. Considering how hard it is to actually get into testing, it makes the most sense just to do it in one sweep. In my daughter's case, the initial testing was done too early to ascertain an accurate ADHD diagnosis. However, if initial testing is done in the elementary years and older, it should be part of the testing, if anything, just to rule out other possibilities.

Epilepsy is a seizure disorder caused by electrical misfires in the brain. It is estimated that a third of all autistic individuals have epilepsy, and seizures are the most common neurological complication of autism (Khan, 2017). I am obviously one of these individuals. Of all the comorbidities, this is the one that scares me the most for my children. For one, they are at increased risk simply because I have a history of seizures. Most importantly, mortality is increased overall with individuals who have epilepsy, including those from external causes such as drowning and Sudden Unexpected Death in Epilepsy (SUDEP) (Robertson et al., 2015). This is why I see the information on Neurofeedback to be especially insightful and hopeful. This is also why I try to take significant steps to maintain my overall health and prevent what triggers I can. My seizures have luckily been controlled by these steps, but unfortunately, that is not always the case, and my heart goes out to the many individuals and families who struggle with this on a daily or frequent basis.

Depression and anxiety disorders are both very common in autistic individuals, with anxiety being the most prevalent issue. I have heard of autistic individuals who supposedly do not have anxiety, but I have yet to meet one. I want to though, if anything, just ask them what that is like. I often see these two hand in hand, with one feeding the other. Individuals can become depressed over time when they have significantly high levels of untreated anxiety. Both of these can also decrease our daily functioning and increase some of our most troublesome autistic symptoms, such as obsessive behaviors, aggressive behaviors, self-harm, sleep disturbance, and social withdrawal (*Autistica,* 2020). The irony of this is it's very possible that we are as anxious as we are because our brains are not necessarily built for this neurotypical world, and with that knowledge, it's no wonder why we get depressed and often shut down.

Obsessive Compulsive Disorder (OCD) has a high comorbidity with autism. Not all obsessive behaviors in autism are indicative of having OCD. Many autistics stim and have other repetitive behaviors, and their focused interests can often be labeled obsessions; however, these are markedly different than the obsessions and behaviors that occur with OCD. OCD behaviors and obsessions are marked by high anxiety and a compulsive and intrusive need behind them, which controls the individual and keeps them from being fully functional.

According to Meier et al. (2015), individuals first diagnosed with autism had a 2-fold higher risk of a later diagnosis of OCD, whereas individuals diagnosed with OCD had a 4-fold higher risk of being later diagnosed with autism. In these cases, it is important to have the OCD properly treated by a medical professional as it can progressively get worse without treatment and increase the likelihood of major depression, severe anxiety, panic disorder, agoraphobia, and/or complete shutdown.

Ehlers-Danlos syndrome (EDS)/hypermobility spectrum disorders (HSD) is a group of 13 heritable connective tissue disorders caused by genetic changes in the connective tissue, with each type having its own unique features, some of which include joint hypermobility, skin hyperextensibility, and tissue fragility (*What is eds?* 2023). Hypermobility is the most common of them, accounting for approximately 90% of all diagnoses. It requires a genetic test to confirm the diagnosis. There is significant research citing that autism and EDS share considerable phenotypic overlap at various levels, including similarities at the molecular, cellular, and tissue levels, and also share a variety of secondary comorbidities, including neurobehavioral, psychiatric, and neurological phenotypes, such as

ADHD, anxiety and mood disorders, proprioceptive impairment, sensory sensitivities, eating disorders, epilepsy, etc. (Casanova et al., 2020). This diagnosis can often be overlooked by medical professionals. I have had clients detail various symptom indicators that are red flag indicators of this, but due to their lack of an official diagnosis of autism, a medical professional had not considered this, and some of the prescribed initial treatments were actually causing more harm.

The unfortunate truth is autism does make one more likely to possess or develop a number of comorbidities, many of which cause functional issues that autistic people often struggle with. A whole book could be devoted to just those.

Here is a non-exhaustive list of others.
- Eating disorders
- Down Syndrome
- Bipolar or other Mood disorders
- Fragile X Syndrome
- Postural Tachycardia Syndrome (POTS)
- Gastrointestinal symptoms
- Intellectual disabilities
- Sleep problems
- Psychosis and Schizophrenia
- Tourette's syndrome

Most autistics do not need treatment for their autism alone—it is due to the impediments to daily life from comorbidities that treatment is often needed. This treatment is important to manage, as left untreated, many autistic comorbidities will deplete an individual and lead to excessive suffering, with shutdown being the least of one's worries.

SUBSTANCE MISUSE AND PROCESS ADDICTIONS

Long before I was ever diagnosed, I was an addiction specialist. I have a national certification as a Master Addiction Counselor (MAC), and I am state-licensed as an Alcoholism and Drug Abuse Counselor (LADAC). It is another of my focused interests. The irony is in graduate school, I had zero interest in this subject area and thought I wanted to do more marriage and family therapy. What I found, however, was when I was actually doing marriage and family therapy, my anxiety would inevitably increase, especially if there was arguing. I also found that when I worked with clients struggling with substance use or process addictions, I actually found I enjoyed it, and I was actually good at it.

Back in my early to mid-twenties, I found myself at risk for developing a drinking issue. I was actually making an attempt to do things more with coworkers and friends at the time, and I found I was compensating for this increase in social situations and the paradox of the overstimulation of these interactions by drinking. Alcohol as a social lubricant is highly effective but also highly problematic. While I knew I did not enjoy drinking, I did find it was able to let me let go of the anxiety I had around other people. In other words, it helped me mask and be somebody else. It also helped to drown out the general overstimulation in many of these situations.

Over time, however, I noticed my anxiety outside of drinking grew, and my mood decreased. I attempted to seek treatment for my anxiety, and I began taking an SSRI — Prozac. Instead of helping, it caused me the worst insomnia I had ever had. So I stopped taking it. I started distancing myself from those individuals and eventually became pregnant with my middle son, but not before losing two pregnancies through miscarriage back-to-back right before him. During my pregnancy with my son, I developed a strong aversion to the smell of alcohol, which never went away. I have been sober for over 17 years.

I firmly believe much of my aversion has a subconscious layer to it. I absolutely noticed an improvement in my overall anxiety and mood when I stopped drinking. However, I have also had loved ones in my life whose lives have been consistently negatively affected due to alcohol. Over time, I developed a subconscious disgust for the substance. My focused interest and research over the years have only exacerbated that. I am undoubtedly aware that I could have easily developed a significant alcohol misuse issue if I had not stopped drinking when I did.

Statistically, there is a higher chance for autistic individuals to develop an issue with substance use or process addiction. Process addictions are behavioral addictions such as gambling, food, pornography, shopping, internet, or gaming. Autistic individuals are twice as likely to develop addiction issues compared to allistics, and an estimated 1 in 5 teens and young adults receiving substance use treatment may have undiagnosed autism (Miller, 2022). The most commonly abused substances include alcohol, marijuana, opioids, hallucinogens, benzodiazepines, nicotine, cocaine, and amphetamines. (Please note: Medical cannabis is not what I am speaking of when I talk about marijuana in this book. I absolutely know of the benefits of medicinal marijuana, especially for many autistics.)

There are a number of different reasons why autistics are more at risk for developing these issues. The primary one is simply because of the way our brains are wired. Remember how our PFC is affected, and it is our executive control center? Because it is affected, we are more likely to struggle with impulsive behaviors in general, but we are also more likely to have emotional dysregulation issues and use substances to cope with those. David Gray-Hammon (2022) also describes in his book *Unusual Medicine* how he believes that addiction is a state of being, one that arises an unmet support need or a collection of unmet support needs, which I also wholeheartedly agree with. Because of our tendency to be socially anxious, many substances are abused as a means to decrease those negative aspects and help us mask and manage our overstimulating environments. But masking should never be something we, as autistics, should prefer to do. Looking back on my own behavior, I realize that it should have been an indicator to me that something was amiss.

Particularly for those with focus issues, amphetamines can often be abused. And on the other side of that, because of our sleep issues, we are also more likely to abuse substances to help us sleep. Sedative hypnotics are another class of prescribed medication I have to be overly cautious to avoid due to how well they work for my insomnia, but also how highly addictive they can become.

Alcohol is the most commonly abused substance for sleep issues and self-medicating in general. Autistics use it and marijuana the most for anxiety. While the latter of those two is less problematic, it can sometimes lead to an increase in anxiety symptoms when the individual is sober. And with increased use of both of those substances, our ability to cope with anxiety as a whole diminishes. I liken them to a weak dam for water. As we use the substance to cope, it pushes the anxiety back and holds it for a short time, but over time, the substance wears off, and all that anxiety that has been collecting behind it comes rushing out. It feels even more overwhelming than when we first started using the substance. The same can be said for benzodiazepines, which is a highly problematic issue with many autistics.

All three of these substances remove our ability to cope with our anxiety in a natural way. And considering we are already predisposed to anxiety, we are more at risk. I liken our ability to cope with anxiety to a mental muscle. If we never do it without the aid of something, it will atrophy, and our ability to cope will be non-existent. Even benzodiazepines are highly addictive and should only be used on rare occurrences. Many people resist wanting to hear that, but the withdrawal from such medications can lead to increased panic attacks and a host of other painful symptoms that often require medical intervention or detox.

Alcohol withdrawal can be deadly if one has built up a high enough tolerance and requires a medical detox, as withdrawal seizures can be deadly. Marijuana and benzodiazepines have also been abused as a means to cope with sensory overstimulation. Many autistics have taken up harm reduction and, therefore, choose to utilize marijuana since it is non-life-threatening. Ideally, medical cannabis is preferred since it is more regulated and less likely to be laced with other substances that can be life-threatening.

Preferably, my choice would be to legalize individuals to grow their own without repercussion, which would prevent the issue of it being laced. While that is rare, it does happen. One concern that heavy cannabis users need to be aware of is the incidence of Cannabinoid Hyperemesis Syndrome, which includes nausea, vomiting, and severe abdominal pain after heavy use. While this issue is not deadly, it can be very difficult to tolerate, and due to the fact many medical professionals miss it during evaluation, the individuals can be left to suffer unnecessarily. When it is identified, the recommended treatment is generally a very hot shower, which generally alleviates the symptoms.

As described earlier in the section prior to this, autistics are more at risk for co-occurring or comorbid diagnoses. Many individuals use substances as a means to cope with the symptoms of those. Also, because we are more likely to have hyper-focused tendencies, we are at risk of getting drawn into process addictions. These are especially tough because some of these can be healthy behaviors and a good means to decompress if done in a healthy manner. For example, gaming is a very popular hobby for autistics. But they are also one of the most likely ones to abuse it and let it get in the way of functioning, sometimes spending so much time on it that they neglect sleep, food, and hygiene, much less other required activities for living.

Internet and pornography addiction are also big struggles for many autistics, with the latter causing complications associated with erectile dysfunction in some men, intimacy issues in relationships, and preoccupation that often gets in the way of general functioning. I have known individuals to lose their jobs when they are unable to refrain from usage even while at their place of employment.

Shame and guilt can be an impetus for increased substance use. This is consistent with allistic usage as well. However, autistics already can have a higher shame meter than most. The cycle begins with the usage of the substance or, in some cases, a behavior. This leads to the individual feeling shame and/or guilt for using and the other behaviors it can lead to. Because the substance adequately numbs that feeling, albeit briefly, they again turn to it, beginning a vicious cycle of abuse. The only way to stop this cycle is to stop the use of the behavior or the substance. Sometimes, binges can often be a result of an individual getting caught in a shame cycle.

Similar to a shame cycle, an autistic can also get caught in a shutdown cycle of substance use. As symptoms that lead to shutdowns increase, many autistics will use substances or increase process addictive behaviors as a means to cope. Inevitably, this will lead to an increase in the symptoms, and shutdown is more likely to come on quicker as a result. Because shutdown is often unbearable, the individual continues to cope with the negative means. I see marijuana used the most in this instance. And while it is not necessarily physically addictive like other substances, there is a definite psychological addiction. These individuals struggle with stopping the substance even though it is definitely negatively interfering with their lives. Individuals caught in this cycle have the hardest time coming out of shutdown.

Biologically, there has been a link to changes in the striatum, a central region of the brain involved in motivation, pleasure, and habitual behavior (Szalavitz & Spectrum, 2017). As a behavior increases in use, the ventral region of the brain, which is connected to impulsive behavior, switches the action toward the dorsal striatum. The region automates behavior into more programmed patterns, which can be set off by specific cues leading to a compulsion that is difficult to restrain, such as drug abuse or process addictions (Szalavitz & Spectrum, 2017).

It is theorized that autistics may be more prone to getting stuck in this pattern. There is numerous other research that has described various other reasons why autistics are more biologically susceptible to substance use and process addictive behaviors. This topic alone could fill another entire book. If you want to read a worthwhile autistic's lived experience with substance misuse, I would definitely recommend David Gray-Hammond's *Unusual Medicine: Essays on Autistic Identity and Drug Addiction*.

Rejection Sensitive Dysphoria and Perfectionism

Rejection Sensitive Dysphoria (RSD) is among the newer terms that are making the rounds in discussions of ADHD and autism. Similar to the aspect of PDA, it is not currently associated with the DSM and is not a formal diagnosis, and many mental health professionals have still not heard of it. It occurs when an individual experiences an intense or overwhelming emotional injury to criticism or rejection, real or perceived, which triggers an overwhelming negative emotional response (Higuera, 2021).

Individuals who suffer from this describe it as feeling an internal wound deep in their innermost self. Considering dysphoria in Greek means unbearable, the term is accurate in its description of the physical and emotional pain the individual feels they are suffering (Dodson, 2022). The term was coined by Dr. William W. Dodson of the Milton E. Hershey Medical Center and was described as something that was fairly common with those who have ADHD. As more studies are concluded, more researchers are finding this to be a common issue with autistic individuals as well.

These individuals often struggle with poor self-esteem and emotional dysregulation issues, which can often be misdiagnosed as a mood disorder or borderline personality. These issues are amplified after an acute situation that involves real or perceived criticism or rejection. They typically have high anxiety in social settings, which leads them to avoid social settings altogether. This is also why it is often misdiagnosed as a social anxiety disorder or considered just a typical symptom of autism if the person is already diagnosed. It also can lead to other relational issues due to the lack of self-esteem and negative self-talk. Sometimes, there is a fear of failure that may prevent the individual from taking steps to try and better their situation. Examples of this include looking for a new job, furthering their education, or even avoiding getting into a new relationship. On the other hand, some individuals set extremely high expectations for themselves as a means to try and overcompensate for fear of failure.

By its very nature, perfectionism can be a trigger to shutdown or burnout for many, but those with RSD find themselves particularly vulnerable to failures. Even allistic perfectionists individuals are at risk for typical burnout. But what many do not realize is that there is a good portion of autistics that are perfectionists. Autistics already have a tendency to hyperfocus on certain tasks, and they will devote long hours with little to no breaks. Over time, these individuals can slide into the perfectionist category due to their tendency to go all in on tasks, with little to no grace for mistakes, and will ruminate over them extensively (Kluger, 2023). Please note, however, one can definitely be a perfectionist without having RSD.

Individuals with RSD have a hard time letting things go and can find themselves stuck in a perseveration loop regarding criticism or rejections for days. The emotional dysregulation of RSD can lead to meltdowns, but when rumination and perseveration mixed with high anxiety occur for long periods of duration, it can also lead to shutdown and increased social isolation, which can lead to significant functioning issues. Consider this example: An individual with RSD gets held back after one of their college classes, where the professor asks them about their last assignment. The professor makes inferences that it wasn't in line with the individual's normal work. The individual leaves the meeting and spends the next day or so ruminating over the interaction and perseverating over what their professor thinks of them. This causes said individual not to want to attend the next couple of classes out of fear, causing them to fall even more behind. The guilt and shame continue to intensify, and they end up missing other things as well.

Like PDA, eventually, more mental health professionals will become more educated on these topics, which may help with preventing misdiagnosis of something that is not accurate to what is actually going on and unnecessary treatments that follow and don't work. One of the key aspects of treatment for RSD is mindfulness. After educating some of my clients about it, several have found solace in knowing they are not alone with this and that it explains a lifetime of internal and external struggles. The negative self-talk can then be managed by replacing it with knowledge of what's going on in their mind and positive self-affirmations that they will get through this, as they have done before. Cognitive Behavioral Therapy (CBT) can also be especially helpful in identifying certain cognitive distortions that can amplify RSD.

Also, with the knowledge of what it is, they can reach out for support from individuals to get an unbiased view of the situation to see if their RSD may be distorting the situation. If it truly is rejection, support can help the individual talk through the situation. Everyone deals with rejection; the objective is to not let it keep you down. Grow from it and move on as best as you can, but trust me, I know that is easier said than done.

I am certain that rejection is the root of why I was and still am often afraid to ask questions when I am confused. I have a very clear memory of when I was little and was staying at a sleepover at my Sunday School teacher's house. We were all watching TV when I looked over in the corner and saw a stethoscope. I believed I knew what it was. Nowadays, we have plenty of toy versions of these. They are pretty fascinating, especially to a child.

Without thinking, I simply pointed and asked what it was. The next thing I know, I got scolded by my teacher's husband, who firmly told me something along the lines of "Don't mess with that!" The tone was harsh, and the look on his face was also harsh. I also glanced at my teacher and noted she gave him a look of displeasure. But the damage was already done. A heavy shame hit me that made me feel like a bad child. Even now, thinking about this memory 34+ years later brings the shame back with fresh vigor. And thus, I try to avoid ever feeling like that again and simply avoid asking questions. Logically, I realize that 99% of individuals will not respond as he did. But there is still always a chance in my mind, and I would just rather try and figure things out if I can.

SHUTDOWN IN CHILDREN

Much of this book addresses autistics of all ages. But I did want to highlight how autistic shutdown specifically affects children since it can often look different than in adults and teens. One of the biggest challenges for autistic children is their lack of autonomy in every facet of their lives. They are told what to do and how to do it in their homes and educational environments. Many have difficulty forming their own self-reliance because if they struggle with communication, many parents and caretakers assume they are not capable and, therefore, do many things for them.

One might be thinking, "How can a child not like someone doing stuff for them, and why would that matter in terms of shutdown?" If an individual has met a neurotypical 2 to 4-year-old they will quickly notice that child wants to do all the things themselves. Even MADtv had a skit devoted to this personification. Stuart is the embodiment of the strong, independent child with his classic retorts of "watch what I can do" and "let me do it," even to his own mother's behest to do what she says. Of course, he typically rebels and does what he wants regardless, and his relatively large size prevents adults from always stopping him. Now imagine if that child is autistic and they are either nonspeaking or minimally speaking. That drive for autonomy still exists, only now they are not as able to express their self-determination aside from meltdowns and refusals. And sadly, they are often seen as less capable because of their many meltdowns, which neurotypicals often mistakenly correspond to this behavior with "low-functioning." It's only years later when many of these children finally find a communication method that helps them to finally show the world what is under their iceberg, that people are finally able to learn they were mistaken about them all along.

If you are not autistic, can you imagine how exhausting it might be to live like this? To not be seen or heard for who you truly are. You rarely get your own desires met because you cannot express them, and sometimes when you do, those around you often refuse. And then add on all those meltdowns you have because of this frustration and some from sheer exhaustion because most children will typically meltdown when they are exhausted. And that is often what shutdown and burnout look like in children. It is lots and lots of meltdowns from not being understood.

This world is not generally built for autistic children. Our schools are designed for the neurotypical child who can sit still with calm bodies, quiet hands, and direct eye contact. False narratives are being taught that these are what help children to learn the best.

Even with IEPs, 504s, and more neurodiversity-informed educators, we are barely scratching the surface of these children's needs. We push therapies that try to make them fit the norm and align with more neurotypical behavioral standards, like Applied Behavioral Analysis (ABA). Despite recent research finding nearly half (46 percent) of those exposed to ABA met the diagnostic threshold for PTSD, and extreme levels of severity were recorded in 47 percent of the affected subgroup, Psychologists and educators still push it (Kupferstein, 2018). This Kupferstein research study (2018) also found respondents of all ages who were exposed to ABA were 86 percent more likely to meet the PTSD criteria than respondents who were not exposed to ABA, and adults and children both had increased chances (41 and 130 percent, respectively) of meeting the PTSD criteria if they were exposed to ABA.

And yet, rather than understand why this occurs, the answer for many ABA providers is to change some of their approaches and call it "new ABA". I am sorry, but no therapy should be a part or full-time job. Not even play therapy, for which I am a Registered Play Therapist (RPT) and a huge advocate. For one huge reason: it doesn't allow for a child to have enough free play, which is how they learn about their environment the best.

We expect many of these children to go to school a full day and then come home straight to this therapy for anywhere from 10, 20, to 40 hours per week. That amount is unnecessary and overly excessive. I get exhausted just by the idea of it. Unfortunately, as I previously described in Part 1, I have had to have ABA training with a past certification that I let lapse and that I no longer support.

But I did learn something. That it is every bit as awful as I initially thought it was. That and the fact that we put these children through operant conditioning, which is similar to dog training, for these many hours in a week is ridiculous.

And despite the research and many adult autistics speaking out against such therapies, we still have many educators and professionals pushing it. Dr. Robert Jason Grant, the founder of AutPlay, stated the problem perfectly when he said, "When those from a neurodivergent identity tell you something does not work for them, tell you what you need, tell you certain things actually hurt them, and ask you to listen to them, and you (not of that identity), ignore what they say, think they cannot know what they need because they are neurodivergent, and decide you know what is best for them, that is what ableism looks like. If you don't know the effects of ableism, here are some: low self-worth, feeling devalued, self-hate, identity struggles, depression, anxiety, attachment issues, and trauma. Listen and do better (Grant, 2023)!"

This is not just a struggle for children who are non-speaking or minimally speaking; this issue extends to autistic children with excellent verbal skills. They also struggle to find autonomy in most of these settings and are frequently pushed beyond the limits that they can handle. They are also at risk for meltdowns due to these same struggles. When parents actually try to change the system for their children, they get a lot of pushback from those in educational and professional settings, sometimes even when the parent is a professional.

I saw this firsthand with my daughter. This child loved school and her teachers. However, this past year in third grade, she began having more and more meltdowns. More and more often teachers were calling us to come and get her. One time, I came and saw her through a window melting down, and many teachers and administration were surrounding her in a room that was locked. My amygdala immediately flipped. I told them, when they finally unlocked the door, that this was not acceptable and that I had previously stated in a meeting that she doesn't need an audience during a meltdown—no one does! They were trying to show her some kind of skills lesson on the board in the middle of this. It is like they do not understand the brain when it is outside of the window of tolerance, especially during a meltdown. Yet, these are the professionals and educators working with her.

Despite my many previous statements that we were opposed to ABA, they again tried to tell us that it was their recommendation in so many words. I later wrote a long email about my stance in writing and why, citing research, putting to rest this topic once and for all. Their next step was to request a Functional Behavior Assessment (FBA). I have my issues with these, but let me be clear when I say they will never see what's under the iceberg. They look for the obvious acute triggers. They don't see the build-up of mistrust, the slow decline over time in mood, and they will never show shutdown or burnout in a child, which was what was driving her behaviors. We made the decision as a family to pull her from public school and homeschool her. Despite my initial ambivalence, it was the right decision for my child, as she is currently thriving.

My child was suffering from shutdown, and I did not even know the extent until after we pulled her. This child, who once loved school, rarely asked about it afterward. The child who never wanted to go anywhere after school all of a sudden started asking to go places. Meltdowns decreased almost completely, and when they did occur, they were short in duration and had an obvious trigger. She completed more schoolwork in one hour each day than she did in almost a full week of school. She enjoyed free play throughout the day, and she began flourishing because of it.

We started her in play therapy with a play therapist colleague of mine, who also works great with this population, to help prevent further dysregulation with all the changes and slowly supplemented it with equine therapy. This child, who typically is fearful of most animals, happens to love horses. We eventually got speech therapy going in our home with another speech therapist family friend of ours and the first person to ever work with her on her speech when she was under two years old. Even her pragmatic speech was making improvements before we started back the speech therapy because of all the free play she was able to do.

On Tuesdays, between her play and equine therapy, we have aquarium time at a new aquarium zoo that recently opened in our area. On days I see clients, I have my older daughter or a part-time nanny, who brings her little daughter to watch her, and she looks forward to them both. We may incorporate Occupational Therapy (OT) back in eventually, depending on her needs. Currently, we have increased her sensory spaces with everything we can think of at the moment. We carefully weigh the demand for another therapy with the potential benefits that it can bring. OT is an amazing therapy though, and one I highly advocate for. Even with all these changes, which can sometimes be difficult to make, my daughter is back to her joyful, silly self.

Sadly, I am fully aware that most situations can not be resolved like ours. Many neurodivergent families have found homeschooling to often be the best fit for their autistic children, but many families do not have that option. I do realize there are some great schools out there. I feel hers was for a long time, but over time with change after change in administration and other things, it no longer fit her needs. We had a child in that school for 16 years straight, so we saw a lot of changes over time. There are some private school options in this area, but those options wouldn't have fit our family logistics—even if they did, they would have been a very costly gamble to hope they were a good fit for her needs.

The only other option for us would have been to keep her in there and fight tooth and nail for every little thing—A fight that many parents have to perform every day. And yes, this is a fight that is necessary to make the changes that need to occur on a systemic scale. I am choosing to use my efforts in this fight on the therapy, advocacy, and writing side of it. But progress on this issue needs to be fought on all sides. So, for you parents who are fighting in the trenches to advocate for your children in schools, I see you and admire you fully. Hopefully, this world will make the changes it needs to be more suitable for our autistic and other neurodivergent children. And if you feel the task is too daunting, look into getting an advocate for you and your child to attend all IEP/504 meetings, because that was going to be my next option. And if you are still not being heard, look into disability lawyers. They are often the big guns that these fights need.

CHAPTER EIGHT

OVERCOMING SHUTDOWN

To a certain extent, shutdowns are an inevitable part of the autistic lived experience. Something we must keep in mind, however, is that shutdowns in and of themselves are not inherently bad. They are a built-in protection mechanism, protecting us from a number of things. More harm can come from an acute, intense meltdown than a typical shutdown of a short duration. Sometimes, acute shutdowns are our warning system that something is amiss. Look at them like the yellow light to warn and meltdowns as the red light to stop. If we keep pushing past these signals, it can be detrimental, allowing chronic shutdown, or burnout, to occur. For some autistics, this chronic shutdown or burnout can last months or even years. It's during these times that we are pouring from empty cups, or as often stated in the neurodivergent community, "You've got no spoons left."

Spoon Theory

If you are an avid social media user and have been a part of any autistic-led spaces, you will probably have noted the term "spoons"— probably in the context of "I don't have the spoons for this today." Spoon Theory was a term coined by Christine Miserandino, which describes the idea of limited energy, using "spoons" as a unit of energy. This measurement is particularly popular with people dealing with chronic illness (Schultz, 2019) and has become a very popular notion in the autistic community to describe our energy capabilities on a given day or time. As the story goes, Christine described to a friend that for individuals with chronic illness, energy is limited and depends on different factors, including stress levels, sleep quality, and pain levels, and depending on these variables, any given day can take away our spoons or energy capabilities (Schultz, 2019). Like those with chronic health illnesses, autistic individuals' spoon capacities are different each day. For many of these individuals they are not always in tune with pushing past spoon capacity until it is too late.

A good example of this occurred during a week in winter when we had an almost full week of ice in our area, preventing many of us from leaving the house for many days. I am not the best at being cooped up, but I managed and made the most of my time doing telehealth, writing, and working out, along with my other family duties. Come Thursday, when it was starting to thaw, I was able to drive. I headed to the office with a shovel and some chemicals in hand. I spent over an hour and a half treating the walkway around our office and then shoveling off all the ice from it. I kept watch of my heart rate on my Fitbit as I am firmly aware of the dangers of shoveling snow, which can cause some heart attacks. And this was ice! I was definitely getting a workout in, but I felt okay, and it never went terribly high, especially compared to my runs that I do. I felt "okay" and kept pushing to get all of it done that I could. I did not want anyone coming into the building and slipping.

When I was done, I headed inside and sat in my chair in my office. I suddenly felt more out of it than usual. I knew right then I would be paying for it later. The next day, I was sick, not with a cold but with what felt like a severe malaise that came with the flu. I even had a low-grade fever. I was like that for three days, and for those three days, my normally very low heart rate measured a good 15+ beats higher than normal. I don't get sick that much. This affected me in everything I needed to do, and I only did the bare minimum required for those three days. I know many are saying that I should have known doing that to myself would wear me out. Let me also point out that aside from roller derby in the past, I have run many races in the past few years, including 5k's, 10k's, 15k's, half-marathons, and even one marathon. Not even after the full marathon did I feel like this. I went past my spoons, BIG TIME! And I paid the price. I was hit with a physical shutdown.

Pushing past our physical capabilities is not the only thing that uses up our spoons. In fact, it is probably more accurate that autistics use most of their spoons to complete executive functioning tasks. We also require a significant number of spoons for social settings and situations, managing our sensory environments, focus, and communication. Our spoon drawer for these tasks is different each day. Today was a good example of my drawer having the spoons needed to accomplish many tasks I had on my list, but it required me to plan in advance and make sure I went to bed really early, which is not always easy for me, but because I was exhausted, I was luckily able to.

Today, my spoons were able to get me through two appointments for my daughter, one trip to a local aquarium, an appointment of my own, insurance credentialing applications, and grabbing dinner on the way home for my youngest three because my husband had his own work thing tonight. I even had some spoons left to write about them. But I assure you, this isn't always the case. I often dread days like these because I have a feeling I will need to cut something because my spoon capacity is low, and I have to cut personal tasks out of my day. These are not usually ones for the kids or clients, which I manage to push through.

Managing our spoon drawer is essential! It is basically practicing self-care on a daily basis. Some things that are part of our daily basic hygiene that are also considered a part of our self-care take spoons. Taking a shower is a great example of this. It takes a good deal of effort and energy some days, but I find once I get it out of the way, I feel much better for it. It's definitely one of those things you have to give some to get some, and some days, you don't even have the bare minimum. Giving yourself grace is a big deal when it comes to spoons. If you don't have them, don't beat yourself up. Ask for help or even delegate if you need to. There is even a group on Facebook for people to ask others for help with spoons. Just look up "Extra Spoons (executive dysfunction & mental illness support & mutual aid)" if you are interested.

Whatever you do, do not ignore your spoon capacity. Try to note them as best you can. If you continue to push past your limit, you will pay the price, just as I did with the ice. Completing a task for the sake of completing it doesn't really help if it costs us too much for it. We live in a society and culture that glorifies overworking and doing it all, but it's costing us too much with too little benefit. I am told on occasion that I do a lot. What people don't see is the rest behind it. I love my rest, and I try to prioritize it as best as I can. I don't try to keep it a secret, but it is definitely the biggest resource that I utilize to get my spoons.

AUTISTIC EMPATHY

One of the most maddening stereotypes of autism includes the fallacy of autistic individuals not having empathy. In 2012, after the horrors of Sandy Hook occurred, many so-called professionals suddenly emerged, pushing disparaging narratives of an autistic's inability to feel empathy as being the reason Adam Lanza committed such a heinous act. They overlooked the numerous family systemic issues and went straight to the fact that he was autistic as being the obvious reason why he did what he did. This was not the first time that disabilities such as autism and other mental health issues have been used as a scapegoat reason for gun violence, and sadly, it will not be the last. The sad truth of this is that "individuals with disabilities of all kinds are more likely to be the victims of gun violence, 2.5 times more likely to be the victims of a violent crime such as robbery or sexual assault, and are more likely to have deadly force used against them by the police" (ASAN, 2023). Despite the rhetoric during these crimes aimed at disabilities being the probable cause, the sad fact is most crimes are committed by people without disabilities.

Much of the confusion and misrepresentation of this fallacy comes from the fact that some autistics struggle with alexithymia. According to research, it is estimated that approximately 50% of autistic individuals have alexithymia (Kinnaird et al., 2019). This condition makes it difficult for some to understand and articulate their emotions; It is not that they are not feeling them. For some of my clients, this manifests in being able to label what they are feeling, especially those emotions that are often very mixed. I myself have struggled with a bit of this in the past when I couldn't put into words the feelings I was having after I took my daughter out of public school. I finally went through a long list of difficult emotions and finally came to terms with the fact that ambivalence was what I was feeling. The emotions themselves were very raw. It wasn't that I couldn't feel them. It was simply difficult to put them into words.

What I have noted, and many autistics have also been clear to point out, is not only do most autistics have empathy, but many of them have highly attuned affective empathy. Affective empathy is the ability to feel what others are feeling. This may be due to what I described in the chapter on masking when I discussed somatic empathy. This is empathy that occurs on an internal autonomic level. The individual may feel what the other individual is feeling, but due to possible alexithymia, they may be having difficulty processing it. My daughter is a great example of this. Since she was really little, she would get very upset if someone around her was upset. Sometimes, she would react in anger because they were upset, which made the other person very confused. Even now, at nine years old, when she hears a baby cry, she immediately asks, "What's wrong?" and has been known to run across a store to try and find the baby to see what the issue is. If someone raises their voice, she immediately asks them how they are feeling, and if they say angry or sad, she will tell them to be happy and becomes upset if they continue to be upset. She doesn't want them to be unhappy and understands emotions enough to understand which ones are pleasant and which ones are not.

Because many autistics have high affective and somatic empathy, they can often find themselves feeling overwhelmed and even more drained from being around people. Even those who are considered extroverts can feel drained after a while because it takes a toll on them to constantly feel what others around them are feeling. This is one reason why I have to limit the number of individuals I work with within a given day or week. I will eventually lose effectiveness if I push myself to see too many clients, which is not good for me or for them. This is also one-way autistic empathy can lead to a shutdown and why some autistic individuals choose to be alone a great deal of the time.

One form of empathy that "some" autistics struggle with is cognitive empathy, also known as the Theory of Mind (ToM) or perspective-taking. To be fair, there are many neurotypical individuals that also struggle with this. Many autistic individuals, myself included, can actually be more adept at this than many neurotypicals and may just do it in different ways (Aucademy, 2022). When cognitive empathy disconnects occur, the neurotypical or autistic individual is not able to cognitively put themselves in the situation of another, resulting in an inability to interpret others' beliefs, intentions, and emotions to be able to interact in socially "normative" ways (Brewer et al., 2017). One example that I have seen some struggle with is when they don't recognize how something they said or did come across as hurtful when that was not their intention. When you try to get them to understand why the other person is upset, they struggle because if someone had done it to them, they would not necessarily have gotten upset. It is not from a lack of empathy.

This often comes down to the literalness of the situation. If they break something of the others and they do not see that thing as important, it is hard for them to connect to that emotion the other is feeling. However, I have found when I can change the object of the situation to match that of something the individual does, in fact, hold dear, they can often connect how they would feel if someone broke that thing which they highly regarded. In short, I have found that ToM can be taught to an extent. It might take repetition over time, but eventually, the concept can often be grasped. It is clear that when this happens, it is generally an issue of understanding, not an actual attempt at causing harm or even a desire to do harm. Again, it can occur in neurotypicals and allistics as well. In fact, I often find neurotypical individuals less likely to be interested in understanding how something they did or said may come across as hurtful, and in cases like that, I end up having vicarious shame or embarrassment for them.

One aspect that often correlates with ToM is the Double empathy problem. This is the notion that two individuals, both of whom are empathetic, come from two different worlds of thought and may not agree on an issue because they cannot see it from the other's perspective. To each of these individuals, their perspective comes from a place of empathy and logic, and they just don't see the other person's perspective and how they would come to that notion. This has been an issue in our home and the cause of many struggles over the years.

This can be especially complicated when the issue is between an autistic individual and a neurotypical one. Often, the issue is that neurotypical people lack the capacity to empathize with autistic people because of their unique social communication style, which can be misinterpreted by neurotypical people, leading to an unfavorable perception of autistic people (Mitchell et al., 2021). This is why many autistics have stated they are drawn to friends who are also autistic. They simply feel more understood, can be themselves without judgment, and are less likely to become the scapegoat if a negative situation arises.

Another term that relates to ToM and cognitive empathy is mindblindness, which is described as an inability to attribute mental states such as desires, thoughts, knowledge, and intentions to self and others and to make sense of and be able to predict another person's behavior (Baron-Cohen, 1995). This term parallels mindreading, and once again, autistics are placed on the side of deficits because "they" are the ones who supposedly do not understand how others can have their own thoughts, plans, and points of view. However, the authors of this term and idea fail to note how neurotypical or allistic people also often lack this ability when they are conversing with autistic individuals, and they cannot see how the autistic individual might have their own thoughts, plans and point of view that differs from theirs.

For many years, autistic voices have been suppressed by "professionals in the field" with no lived experience educating the world about the many supposed social and communication deficits of autistics. Now that autistic voices are making themselves heard and are disputing many of the old stereotypes and out-of-date notions that have been used against them, they are getting a lot of pushback. Many are being gaslit with statements such as "You can't be autistic if you have empathy" or "If you were really autistic, you wouldn't be saying that." It's exhausting to always have to plead incessantly to be heard. While many professionals are starting to listen and learn from this, others who are stuck within the deficit-disability model are still too proud and arrogant to acknowledge they came from a place of misinformation and were misguided.

In opposition to the out-of-date deficit-disability model is the social disability model, which explores the disability of autism resulting from disadvantages bound to social construction and cultural norms (Chapple et al., 2021). It is this model and notion that has pushed the movement of the neurodiversity paradigm, which has taken the offensive scapegoating over the years and turned it into a human rights movement for those with neurologically atypical conditions. This paradigm follows the view that all human brains and resulting perceptions differ to a degree (Milton, 2020). If we view this in the context of the double empathy issue, we can see how two individuals, regardless of their neuro-differences, can come to two different points of view, and neither is necessarily incorrect. Systemically, the stereotyping and stigmatizing views towards autistic people are contributing further to socio-communicative breakdowns that are the primary component of the double empathy problem (Chapple et al., 2021).

The emotional labor it takes for autistics to constantly have to carry the weight of being perpetually equated to being deficient and incapable of empathy or understanding of others' points of view is beyond exhausting and continues to take its toll on every ounce of our being. Some days, we just don't have the spoons to fight. Many days, we push well past our limit of spoons and pay the price of that in the days following. On those days, we often refrain from social media as a means to protect ourselves, but it can also affect our daily functioning in our families and places of employment. Many autistic advocates find that their advocacy leads to significant shutdowns. Sadly, this fight shouldn't be this hard, but we do all have the hope that reaching that goal one day of being seen as equal, whatever our differences, will be well worth it. However, we still have a long way to go before we get there.

ADDRESSING SHUTDOWN

So far, this book has elaborated in length on the many ways autistics can get to a shutdown. I am certain there are definitely more triggers as well. It's good to be able to name a state that we are in and what's going on when we are there, but we need to understand how we got to that point in the first place. The key to prevention is mindfulness. While not all shutdowns can be prevented, we are capable of seeing it coming from a distance. We must learn from our own experiences and past struggles with it and identify our own behavioral patterns.

Importance of Rest and Self-Care

So, your battery is depleted, or your energy is quickly diminishing, and whether it is showing on the outside of your system, you are definitely feeling it internally. The importance of rest and decompression cannot be overstated. Depending on the severity of the situation and the significance of the depletion, each individual needs to plan out a route of decompression. That route will look different for everyone. If you are generally just in the lethargic and malaise stage and able to push through your basic daily requirements, be on the lookout for decompression periods and start planning your rest. Often, short bursts of rest can help to give a second wind of energy. This can be as simple as a short nap. Research has even shown that a simple 20-minute nap can show considerable benefits by improving sleepiness, performance level, and self-confidence in task performance and suppressing EEG alpha activity during eyes-open wakefulness (Hayashi et al., 1999).

If you are like me, however, short naps can be difficult because I am not able to fall asleep quickly. There have been a few occasions that I have a late cancellation and set my phone alarm for 45 minutes in hopes of getting a few minutes of that in some restful sleep, and it has done wonders for me when I can. Another option to consider, even if you have just a few minutes available, is a simple Leg-in-chair yoga post that is great for calming your mind and your nervous system and can improve mental function, including concentration, memory, and processing abilities (Lailin Yoga, 2019). This is not a good pose for those with high blood pressure, heart conditions, glaucoma, or back or neck issues. And as always with anything physical, you want to check with your doctor, even for gentle yoga poses, just to rule out the possibility of any risk.

This pose requires a chair or couch, which is what you will be laying your calves on as you rest on the floor. Positioning your body so that the thighs are at about a 45° angle to the body, place the calves on the seat of the chair but have the knees off the edge of the seat. Let your hands rest by your side and rotate the palms and the insides of the elbows to the ceiling to open through the chest and draw the chin towards the chest to lengthen through the neck (Lailin Yoga, 2019). I often do this between sessions on my floor in my office on my super soft rug and use my ottoman for my legs. I typically use a throw pillow for my head. This move also helps with boosting immunity and improving circulation (Lailin Yoga, 2019). It's not a nap, but this pose has a lot of great benefits that can help you feel as though you got some rest and is a great self-care method. Yoga itself has been known to have many therapeutic effects.

I also look forward to being able to sleep in on occasion. Because I am a natural night owl, it helps knowing I can sleep in the next day and unwind more at night. Everyone's sleeping in looks different, and even my own has changed over the years, and I am not able to sleep as late as I once could. But I still look forward to not having any morning demands, not having to rush around, and being able to just lay in bed when I wake up and chill to my heart's content. For some, this may be sitting on their couch undisturbed, watching TV or reading a book, and drinking some coffee or other calming beverage. The undisturbed part is very important! It is not really self-care or rest if you have demands or distractions around you.

Self-care is the best way, in general, to recover from shutdown or imminent burnout. It's also the best time to do all the soothing stims that you want. They are free, and you are able to do them in just about every setting. I even have some for when I am in a session that doesn't distract my clients at all. In every session, I do have a large hand-knit blanket on me that I have made that I enjoy for both light pressure and hand stimming. My office also has stress balls and small animal hand squishes for myself and clients to use if needed. The rug I mentioned earlier is one of the softest rugs you will ever feel, and some clients like to take their shoes off and feel it.

There are some other great methods of self-care that I highly recommend, but some of them do cost money. Massages are one of my utmost favorites. I have monthly massages but would get more if my schedule allowed. For me, this is a great way to meet my light pressure and nap needs because it is inevitable I will nod off during them. I do not do Swedish or deep-pressure massages, but there are those who really like those. My massage therapist also uses aromatherapy, and I get to choose the oil she uses before each session. There is a stress-scented one that I absolutely love. Reflexology is another great self-care treatment I use. I am lucky in that I rent an office to an individual who is a reflexologist right across the hall from me, and she is amazing. I try to get at least one every week, but sometimes my schedule makes that difficult. I typically fall asleep during those as well.

One treatment of self-care I have not tried but have an interest in is float tanks or sensory deprivation tanks. There are some places in our area that offer them. These 1-hour floats are great ways to utilize mindfulness and have been known to help with anxiety, sensory overwhelm, focus and concentration issues, pain, and cardiovascular health. Research has shown that stress, depression, anxiety, and intense pain were significantly decreased, whereas optimism and sleep quality increased in those who utilize floatation therapy (Kjellgren & Westman, 2014). Some individuals have reported having hallucinations while floating, which can be attributed to extreme sensory deprivation and has nothing to do with an actual symptom of psychosis. However, this may be a deterrent for some. If you still enjoy the water but are not interested in float therapy, sometimes a simple hot bath or shower can do wonders. Other types of self-care treatments include acupuncture or chiropractic care.

Other methods of self-care that do not cost anything include guided meditation or imagery. There are some great ones you can find on YouTube with beautiful imagery and music. There are also several self-care apps that offer these, but some include a fee for extra offerings, but they can still be very useful. Another one I like to do when the weather is nice is going outside. The outdoors has a lot of options for self-care. Hikes, even light ones, are very therapeutic. Our area in Northwest Arkansas has a lot of hiking opportunities, and it is also rich in walking trails for those who prefer leisure strolls, biking, or running. Trail running is a big thing in this area as well, and it is my preferred mode of running. We just have to be careful and watch for certain wildlife, like snakes, that can be problematic at certain times of the year. Having grown up near the woods as a child, I still turn to nature as one of my favorite coping tools. If you live in a city, a remote park can do wonders.

These above-described interventions are great ways to address acute shutdown or even prevent it. However, if you have been in shutdown for a long time and are getting to the point where it is becoming depressed or worse, you need a more intense approach to recovery. Think of this situation as an intense illness that needs addressing because, for all intents and purposes, it is—So much so that those with resources, such as celebrities, often will admit themselves into an acute treatment center for "exhaustion." Granted, many of these instances are a lot more complicated than that, but the idea is not a bad one. Sometimes, you need an intense approach to remove yourself from all distractions and get away from all environments that have led to you getting to this point.

It does happen for some that this extreme shutdown has already led to major depression that often has suicidal thoughts, psychosis, or other symptoms attached to it. In those circumstances, acute hospitalizations can do wonders if the place is a quiet, restful place. However, if it is not, issues may become worse if it doesn't give the rest and quiet an individual needs to recoup. This is the type of shutdown that is imperative to try and prevent as much as possible, as the outcome can be deadly for an autistic. Once you have been to this point, you never want to let yourself get to it again.

When I feel on the verge of a shift in my shutdown and my short bursts of rest and self-care are not quite as helpful as I need, I go for my "big guns," which are scheduling a weekend getaway or just time away. As I described in the first part of this book, those often look like a weekend stay at a cabin, lake house, or somewhere I can be undisturbed with no demands and as little human interaction as possible. The goal of those stays is to rest and sleep how I want to, in peace and quiet and get back to knowing myself. I also try to reach a point where I crave being with others again. If I can get to that point, I know I am refueling as I should.

Cost can often be an issue that prevents an individual from utilizing this. Sometimes, even asking a friend if you can come to stay and "get away" can be better than staying where you are, especially if there are a lot of demands and sensory overwhelm. Try and choose a friend who has a low sensory environment, and the more privacy that you can get, the better. Tell them you are not looking to be entertained but literally to decompress and get away. I know this can be difficult for some individuals with limited friends and support in general. The next best thing would be a no-cost camping trip, even if it is in your vehicle. Desperate times call for desperate measures sometimes. But if you can find a nice quiet space in nature, this could do wonders for you.

If I am not quite to the point of needing no human interaction, I may plan a retreat or a camping trip with some loved ones. Those can definitely be refreshing to the soul and sometimes can help curb the cost that can be associated with staying in places like hotels, Vrbo, Airbnb, and cabins. Some individuals have even gone so far as to schedule a time at a retreat center or monastery. And if a weekend is not long enough, plan for longer. While these may sound like vacations, the difference is they may need to occur on a regular basis, and the point is not to site-see but to just "be." I guess for me, vacations are often exhausting, and I need a decompression time after those, but that is typical because I have my family with me, and most of what I do, I am doing for them. No demands, rest, and limited or no distractions are the points of these "big gun" methods.

The ultimate "big gun" method would be on the lines of taking a leave of absence (LOA) or sabbatical. This can be done from either a job or from an educational setting. Sometimes, this is done when someone is between jobs, and the individual is not ready to jump right into another job. This, unfortunately, is not an option for many, however, which is why many individuals get to a state of shutdown in the first place. Most of the time, it is avoided due to the financial constraints that many individuals struggle with, a significant number of them living paycheck to paycheck.

For these individuals who feel their job is playing a significant role in their shutdown, I advise them to look into seeking another job. I know change can be difficult, and applying for new jobs requires spoons, but staying in a job that is increasing the symptoms of shutdown will eventually cause one to either have a health issue requiring treatment and an inability to work or, in some cases, lose the job altogether.

Another reason that prevents individuals from utilizing an LOA is the sheer notion that many employers or educational institutions are not supportive of it. Several cultures really struggle with this notion and attach shame to measures such as this, which really needs to change. But if it is an option that one can take, it can sometimes be the difference between shutting down or avoiding burnout altogether. Sometimes, this much-needed time off can produce motivating clarity for the individual, which allows them to realign their priorities in the first place.

Preventatively, one aspect to keep in mind is utilizing mindfulness when your calendar has a particularly busy season coming up. Every week on my calendar vacillates in the number of demands that are going to be required. If I have a particularly busy week with high demands coming up, I schedule the weekend prior to being what I call bare minimum days. These include minimum demands for social and physical output of any kind. As a runner, I liken them to tapering right before a big race. The goal is to get as much rest as you can prior to all your obligations so you go into it as refreshed as possible. Ideally, I would like about five days, but I will take what I can get. I am also sure to schedule rest at the end of the week for recovery.

For children in shutdown, it might seem like a simple suggestion to prescribe naps, and while those are definitely not a bad idea, many children are not always keen on taking them. This is especially so for those who don't normally take them. This is the case for my daughter. She will not take one, no matter how hard I try to get her to. Rest is still encouraged, however, even if done through different means. Decompression can come in the form of watching TV, playing on a tablet, or other types of gaming. Free unstructured play of any type is good for decompression and rest.

I have known some parents to take a mental health day from the school where the child will have no demands placed on them. Some make it a day all about the child and take them for ice cream, park play, and other fun things of the child's choosing. I think this is a great idea and can definitely help a child who is in the earlier stages of a shutdown. Perfect attendance should not be the goal when a child is barely staying afloat! It can also be used sporadically to prevent a shutdown.

Unfortunately for my daughter, she was well into a deep shutdown, and we were only able to help her after pulling her out of public school. Even the idea of having fun days on weekends or going for fun treats sporadically was too much for her during the worst of it. She needed substantial rest and low demands to be able to get back to baseline. And PDA children are more likely to need preeminent plans for rest and decompression. But I cannot advocate enough for unstructured free play and fewer scheduled activities. Other mindful activities that can also be included on a daily basis are coloring, sensory or sand play, swinging, or any outdoor play.

Supports

Support systems are a good way to prevent getting to the worst part of the shutdown. While it should be an aspect of prevention, it should also be a big part of the recovery process as well. Some support can be requested through accommodations at work or at school through an IEP or 504. If your work is hesitant to provide accommodations, you may benefit from getting these requested through a therapist or doctor. Sometimes, these need only be temporary, but sometimes, they may be needed on a regular basis. Don't be hesitant to ask or request them, however. If you assume you will not be approved, you have no chance of meeting these needs.

Counseling or play therapy can be a very positive support for many individuals and children. Even if you find it difficult to find a neurodiversity-informed therapist or one that works with autism, look for one that works with exhaustion, compassion fatigue, etc. Even before my official diagnosis, I was able to meet with a therapist who specializes in compassion fatigue in therapists and helpers, and she was a great help, even though she did not understand the autism aspect. Don't be hesitant to try and educate them as well. A good therapist wants to learn from their clients as well—I know I do. And if you don't find one that is a good fit, keep looking. I tell my clients that I am not a perfect fit for all (no one is), and I will not take offense at all if they want to try someone else. I will even help them with other referrals.

I do realize that finding a therapist can be difficult. Many aren't able to accept all insurance, and there are also other variables to consider. I tell many who are seeking a therapist to look at Psychology Today because you can narrow down your search by location, insurance, issues, gender, types of therapeutic modalities, price, ethnicity, faith, sexuality, and ages they work with. Many private practice therapists use this and will keep it updated if they are actively taking on new clients or if they have a waitlist. Using your insurance company is not always an up-to-date means to find a therapist. Most therapists also offer telehealth as an option now, so even if you don't have someone local, you can ideally find a therapist in your state that you can see. I understand that this is vastly different in other countries, and there are complexities that come with each one of them. I can only speak from the experience of my country.

I am not an advocate for those online therapy platforms because many are not HIPAA compliant, and even in their privacy policies, they will tell you they share your information with third parties, which I find unethical. Many also draw you in with promises of varied therapists and specialties and, in the end, cannot deliver, and yet you are on the hook for their monthly fee even if you can't find help. Some even use false advertising that they have specialized therapists whose profile information they have taken from other sources, and then when you try and schedule with them, you are then directed to other therapists that are in their company. They also often pay their therapists very low rates, and, in the end, even if therapists use them as a supplemental income, they typically end up leaving, so there ends up being a high turnover. That means you will have a good chance of having to start all over if you have been with a therapist for a while.

If you want more stability, find a private practice therapist or small group practice. Even large agencies tend to have high turnover. If you do not have insurance, do not let that deter you from seeking help. Many Universities offer low-cost counseling with interns. Many group practices also offer this and charge anywhere from $15-$40 (USD) per session, and they are capable of offering telehealth as well. My practice sometimes has one intern who offers low-cost counseling at $15 per session and some for pro bono. The downside to this offering is that these interns will end up graduating and moving on to other places. A typical period an intern sees clients is 5-10 months. So, there is a turnover of therapists, but most have your information and notes to look at, so it is not quite as daunting to restart. And many issues can be dealt with during that time.

Other means of support include social media groups, a lot of which are autistic-led. Despite this, it can still be challenging trying to find the right one for you. Find the one with the right balance for your needs. Some are not the best to ask questions without judgment, while others are low-key and give great feedback. As I mentioned in the section about spoons, there is even one to help you do a task if you need it. Ideally, you need to find one or more that is supportive for you and not draining. This is true for any social connection that you find. Autistic-led pages can also be a means to find community. The autistic community as a whole can be a vast resource for information and connection.

Discord can also be a good place for individuals to find connections. Just be on the lookout for toxic behaviors that are not beneficial to you, and keep good boundaries. Again, this should be the case for any situations and connections you find in general. Some individuals have found connections through Dungeons and Dragons (D&D) groups and events. The show Stranger Things was really good about bringing that hobby back for many. While groups like these are generally hobby groups, friendships can often be formed, and one can find a source of connection within.

In some cities and areas, there are social groups specific to those who are autistic. Meetup.com can be a great way to find some of those or any group. Community volunteering and churches can also be a means to get involved with a social support system. While the issue of religious trauma has turned some individuals away, there are churches out there that are openly accepting of everyone, and some are non-denominational if that is something that you are seeking.

A social support system is not the only means of coping. Others include idiosyncratic calm hobbies such as arts and crafts of any kind, reading, designing, writing, journaling, music, exercise/sports, photography, etc. Look for something that will help with decompression and has low to no demands. They could be non-thinking activities or creative-minded undertakings. My oldest and middle son are big into creating digital music, which is a great decompression and creative outlet. A good ol' binge-fest of your favorite show and even gaming can be great ways to decompress after long times of being "on." I know that counters what many therapists say, but in truth if balance is maintained, these can be healthy coping mechanisms if they do not get in the way of one's functioning.

I would advise, though, that if you are dealing with high anxiety, it might be best to choose a show or game that won't increase that because there are definitely ones that will. I personally love some good thrillers and horror movies, but there are times that I have to abstain for my own nervous system's benefit. Whatever your thing is, if it's helpful and healthy, do it. Remember those four questions to ask yourself to see if they meet the healthy category. 1.) Is it good for you? 2.) Is it good for others? 3.) Does it make you feel good? 4.) Is it easy to do? The easy part can be subjective. Some might enjoy a bit of a challenging puzzle or something of the like. And that is completely fine.

Sensory Regulation Strategies

I am a lover of all things sensory. Occupational Therapy (OT) without ABA components is one of my most recommended therapies for autistic children and teens. I honestly wish more clinics would provide services for adults, but they are definitely hard to come by. Sensory modulation or regulation has become an important piece in mental health occupational therapy. It is defined as the ability to self-organize and regulate reactions to sensory inputs in a graded and adaptive manner and the ability to self-organize inhibitory and excitatory sensory stimulation and adapt to environmental changes (Brown et al., 2018). If incorporated adequately, it can help autistic individuals to better perform and adapt to various challenges they may face, including shutdown.

Benefits of sensory modulation include increased self-awareness, resilience, self-esteem, and the ability to self-nurture, engage in self-care and social activities, as well as cope with various triggers (Champagne, 2008). More OTs are becoming educated on the importance of sensory practices within the mental health domain, but mental health professionals, unfortunately, are not outside of some valuable play therapy training. Autistic adults are the ones missing out on the benefits of sensory modulation due to a lack of therapeutic knowledge in mental health professionals who work with them because most do not have the training on this topic that is offered to play therapists. Not all play therapists are interested in this topic, but I do feel it is an important one because of the many benefits it can offer.

The good news is many sensory modulation activities can be done in the autistic's own environment and are a great way to prevent and help recover from a shutdown. Some of these activities have been discussed in various parts of this book already, and they include grounding activities, relaxation/calming activities, self-nurturing and self-soothing activities, distracting activities, mindfulness, strategies for identifying and coping with triggers, activities promoting increased connectedness, and environmental modifications (Champagne, 2008). Many are described in the previous portion of this chapter and are great sensorimotor activities.

Other sensory modalities that are helpful include the use of weighted blankets, sound or music therapy, brushing techniques, aromatherapy, light therapy, and pet therapy. One can also develop their own sensory diet that integrates various daily strategies that one can employ as a means to prevent issues. While this incorporates a sensory kit made for yourself, it also includes prevention and crisis strategies and sensory-supportive environments and spaces. You will need to include physical environment modifications such as workspace modifications, sensory room, or sensory-safe modulation places within the home. This can be as simple as utilizing a closet as a safe place to use these sensory modulation activities and find comfort.

My ideal space would include one of those really large bean bags that are so big they can take up a small room and be used as beds. I would have a large, big-screen TV that would have beautiful imagery and light ambient music playing. I would have cozy blankets and one weighted blanket all over me and all the sensory toys within reach I would need. Add in a clean, light scent and some slightly sweet coffee, and this would be my dream sensory environment. And while not all of it is possible right now, I do what I can to get as close to it as possible and make the most of what I do have. Try to transform your environment as much as you can to meet your individual needs.

Gift of Contentment

Over the years of working with clients, one of the most common struggles many have, despite the issue that brought them into counseling, was their desire to find happiness. In the midst of a shutdown, it is common for individuals to struggle to find this said happiness. The reason is that happiness is an emotion, and it is fleeting, much like all other emotions. Instead, I guide clients to try and find contentment. This is more of a choice in having a specific state of mind that, despite their circumstance, they can find joy, pleasure, or even peace in their lives. This has helped me push through some very difficult shutdowns and circumstances.

I have to remind myself that these situations are temporary and to look for the positives in things. I monitor my hope and those thoughts that will fuel or destroy it. I am mindful of those negative thoughts and try to replace them with positives, which is not easy to do and takes a great deal of effort. But positive thinking is a great skill to develop, and it helps to increase mental toughness. This also includes being mindful of those negative influences that can be driving me to more negative thoughts. While this can definitely be people, for me, it is generally influences that are online, such as negative or depressing news. If it is hard for me to go without seeing these during these episodes, I have to limit being online altogether.

More than anything for me, I have to willingly let go of control or at least remind myself that I didn't have it in the first place. This is a hard one for me. I am a fixer by nature and want to fix problems as they occur. For some logistical things, this can be done immediately. But for most things, it's not that easy. When something triggers my anxiety, I want to immediately deal with it so I can get rid of the anxiety. This is definitely tied to my demand avoidance style of staying ahead of demands.

A common way this bites me is when a situation falls into my lap at the end of a business day. The situation is resolvable. However, I am now limited because I am unable to call certain powers because the business day is closed. In the past, this would send me into a meltdown. Now, I am better able to manage them by talking myself through the situation mentally. I literally have to remind myself that I don't have any control over this situation and that I am actually letting it control me. I had to process this and analyze what the real root and fear was behind it. Along with just not having control over the situation, I also have a fear that I will forget the situation if I let it go, and then something even worse will happen. It seemed so simple, yet that fear was controlling my life, so I started to simply schedule a reminder to remind me to address it the next business day and time that I knew I could address it.

That small step helped so much by showing me what little control I did have and still giving me some peace in the situation.

Trying to control every situation will diminish our contentment. We can recognize what areas we do have control in, but we also need to recognize that we cannot control and fix everything. We cannot get rid of a shutdown immediately. We can take active steps to prevent it or even minimize it. But we do not have superpowers that can get rid of them at will. Instead, we need to be able to find joy in the little things and remind ourselves that we can get through this. We might not be happy at this moment but we can find some peace and contentment in the circumstances. We can choose to just "be" and take each day one day at a time.

My Journey to Rest and Recovery

After my diagnosis and the events of 2022, I realized more than ever that my need for rest was at an all-time high. I had been pushing through an exceedingly difficult year and was running way past empty. My tendency to push past 110% had accumulated to a very exhausted, run-down state. Work was going well, but I was having days where I had little to give to people in general. I told my husband that I needed to get away and not have any demands on me or converse with anyone.

Back in 2017, I had a similar feeling. I do not remember the exact happenings prior to that situation, but I remember feeling rundown and needing to get away from people. I had asked my husband about asking his parents in Oklahoma if I could borrow their little cabin in the woods for a weekend so I could do some writing. They did one better and lent me their house while they stayed in the cabin. That weekend, I spent a good majority of it writing. Much of that writing has ended up being part of this, funny enough. I spent the rest drinking coffee and relaxing and made a quick trip to see my parents for a couple of hours. It was exactly what I needed. Unfortunately this time, I did not have the gift of time to logistically plan a trip to Oklahoma and work it out with them. I was in a much more dire state this time.

So, I decided to reach out to my daughter's mother-in-law, who had a lake house that she had offered us to use if we ever needed it. I told her about my struggle, and she understood it well. We scheduled a time that happened to be close to my birthday. I could not have asked for a better birthday present.

I spent the weekend talking to no one. I slept in, sat on the deck, watched lakegoers, and pet the neighbor's dog. I also was able to get some PowerPoint work done on a Neurodiversity-Affirming training I was putting together for two fall training I was leading. This work was not pressing and, therefore, not demanding. It was enjoyable because I was not rushed. I would type, then walk away, drink my coffee, and listen to music. I had no pressure and no demands. It was glorious and just what my mind, body, and soul needed. I did not have to interact with anyone. I even took a short walk to the lake and back. By the end of the weekend, I was back to more of a baseline functioning level. I definitely could have stayed a good week and been completely okay with that, but the weekend sufficed.

When I came back to the world of the living, I felt more at peace. I was even able to take my youngest son to a birthday party at the skating rink at its busiest time. It was overwhelming, but my ability to manage it was stronger. My ability to face all of my other demands was also stronger. I will never feel 100% calm or at peace with demands, but I am able to process and work around or through them to some extent.

This specific time of year comes with birthday planning, as September is generally when we have a combined birthday party for all three of my boys for the family. I was able to jump right into that planning and not feel overwhelmed. This time of year is often very difficult for me, even in a good year. This is when all the kids and Steven start back to school. He is a teacher, so with that comes the end of summer and his ability to get things done that I might not be able to get to. This particular year, he was also in another online master's program himself, so there was even less time he could be available when home.

To add to the usual stress, my youngest was struggling more than usual at school. It was not until later that we found out that they never replaced a paraprofessional who was in her class after they left. It was also later noted that the sensory room she had utilized in the past was made from a grant her Kindergarten year had been cut to bare bones, and she was not even able to use it as needed as a means to prevent her meltdowns.

Marked with increased anxiety at all the recent changes in our family and the changes in her school environment, she was not doing well. I had made the statement to my husband that if things were to continue, I would be making the decision to pull her from school and would be homeschooling her. He really did not like that, and it caused issues at that time. It would not be until later that he also realized that would be the best option for her.

In October, I was doing well but was attempting to see if I could schedule a time to fit a fall break in of some kind. Fall is my favorite time of year, especially in Northwest Arkansas, where the leaves are beautiful. Normally, this time of year, I look forward to a Fall retreat with the ladies from our church. This year, I needed less of a group thing and asked my sister and mother to do something. I also planned a night for myself at a cabin near where we wanted to meet up. There, I was able to get in a long hike just before dark and an extremely hot long bath, which I never get at home. The next day, I met up with my sister and mother and got the essentials before we headed to a nearby Yurt retreat center. There, we spent one full day just talking and the rest of the two and a half days doing several different relaxing things. This was another soul-replenishing endeavor. It was the perfect fall retreat.

The next month consisted of finishing preparations for those two training sessions that were coming up in November. They were both scheduled back-to-back. One was at a state counseling conference, and the next was the week after at a regional counselor meeting. Normally, I struggle at conferences because they are consistently around large crowds. These crowds were not excessive, and I was smart enough to make sure I had my own room for a place to retreat to and turn off at the end of each day. There, I would eat sushi and just be. I would check in with my husband and watch the family on our Google Nest cameras. By the end of the conference, I was ready to go and be back with my family. I did not feel depleted in any way.

When the next training came along, I felt even more comfortable and found I enjoyed presenting, especially on this topic, which is one I can infodump on for a long time.

I had been mentally preparing for these events for several months, and now that they were finished, I even had a moment of "Now what?" I do not even remember the last time I had one of those. This entire year had been filled to the brim with event after event, and now I could just focus and be for a bit. One thing that my brain struggles with, however, is being idle. When it is well rested, I enjoy researching, reading, and doing. I will be like this when I am well into my silver years.

This opportunity allowed me to look at some projects I had placed on the back burner. One of those projects was applying for a Ph.D. program that I had been eyeing for several months. I should back up a bit here. I had mentioned previously that there were other reasons that I had also considered to be important for looking at getting an official diagnosis. One of these was the idea that I eventually wanted to get a Ph.D. to open the door for doing autism or neurodiversity research.

While I had become a particularly good student as an adult, the prospect of completing a dissertation and having to defend it brought about a lot of anxiety. For one, my struggle with pragmatics and word aphasia has increased since I was a young adult and had those seizures. With written expression, I am able to think through my words and put them more concisely than when I am processing them verbally. I am open with my clients about my struggles with finding words at times. But in a Ph.D. program, I needed to have the official diagnosis for accommodations that I may need at certain points. Sadly, self-diagnosis would not have been something that would benefit me in a program like that.

The Ph.D. program is in Change Leadership for Equity and Inclusion, with an emphasis on Community Leadership. I did, fortunately, get accepted into this program. The acceptance came on the same day that my first grandchild was born. My essay included my lived experience and topics of desired research. I feared every day that being open about my diagnosis would be a barrier. This is a fear many autistics have in many things, and that is one thing I am trying to change. Since I was accepted into this program, it will be imperative that I stay on top of my focus and energy expenditures and rest when needed. I did a decent job of this when I did my two master's programs. For me, I know it can be done.

I have learned many lessons throughout this past year on the topic of an autistic shutdown and wish I would have known these things all my life. This has become a focused interest of mine, and I have enjoyed researching and helping many clients work through their own struggles through this. One particular day within the past week, I found that of seven clients I saw in one day, six were autistic, and four of them were dealing with issues of an autistic shutdown, some of them for many months. I realize increasingly how prevalent this issue and struggle is for many.

Final Thoughts

Shutdown is going to be an accustomed part of their lives for many autistics. I am one of those. I know they will come, given how much I put on myself. I definitely am the primary cause of many of my shutdowns. But even so, there are some that occur without my contribution. Managing them is as important as managing any other symptoms, illness, or disability. Because if we don't, they can lead to worsening symptoms and illnesses such as depression. The longer it is left untreated, the more likely it is for that to occur.

An autistic shutdown normally lasts days, but for some, it can last weeks or even months. There are even some autistics who have reported feeling like they have been shutdown for years and they are barely able to meet their daily basic needs. For those, it is going to take a tremendous amount of support to help pull them out.

My hope is that you can use many of the discussed components of prevention and treatment discussed in this book to minimize these shutdowns and be able to live full lives without it keeping you dejected. Open up to others if you have. Reach out for help. It doesn't always have to be counseling, even though that is a great support. Opening up to others that we might be close to, with our vulnerability and struggle, can often bring about the support that may help us as much as rest can. For example, if someone asks you how you are doing, be honest. My daughter's mother-in-law has done this, and I have been open and honest rather than giving the same cliché response of "fine." In doing so, I was able to not only get support, but she was able to even point me in a direction where I could find some rest.

This might require us to break some old patterns of behavior. But some of those behaviors are what led us to this repetitive struggle in the first place. And with any other disability or illness if there is a symptom that causes a lot of issues and we can prevent or manage them, why wouldn't we? The same goes for a shutdown. We can manage and prevent a substantial amount of it. We just need to find what works for us, and that will be a trial-and-error process. But whatever it takes, do not give up. You are worth it, and your life can be significantly more enjoyable because of it.

For those who enjoy worksheets, I have included a shutdown profile in the next section to help outline some of the measures discussed in this book. There is also a section of great resources located at the end of this book, including books, websites, and activists to follow. While I am not able to include them all, this will give you a good start. These are also a good start to initiate support because once you open the door to one of these, more will start being recommended to you that are along the same line of support. Much of this community has been a tremendous wealth of knowledge and support for many autistics dealing with a variety of needs. It is my hope that if you haven't already, you can have the door opened to you for this much-needed support.

SHUTDOWN PROFILE

AUTISTIC SHUTDOWN PROFILE

PRIMARY SYMPTOMS
(CIRCLE YOURS)

LIMITED PATIENCE
DECREASED ENERGY
IRRITABILITY
INCREASED SENSORY SENSITIVITY
DIFFICULTY WITH SIMPLE TASKS
APHASIA (TROUBLE FINDING WORDS)
INCREASED MELTDOWNS
AUTISTIC REGRESSION
STRUGGLING WITH DAILY TASKS
COMMUNICATION STRUGGLES
POOR IMPULSE CONTROL
INCREASED RIGID THINKING
DECREASED WORKING MEMORY
INCREASE IN PHYSICAL STRUGGLES
INCREASED AGGRESSION
INCREASED ANXIETY &/OR PANIC ATTACKS
DEPRESSION
DIFFICULTY LEAVING HOME
DIFFICULTY GETTING OUT OF BED
INCREASED SOCIAL ANXIETY
INCREASED MASKING
INCREASE IN TRIGGERS
INCREASE IN DEMAND AVOIDANCE
INCREASE IN APATHY OR DECREASE IN EMPATHY
INCREASED EMOTIONAL DYSREGULATION

@theautist

AUTISTIC SHUTDOWN PROFILE

PERSONAL TRIGGERS
(CIRCLE YOURS)

●   ●   ●   ●   ●   ●

OVERTHINKING

TRAUMA

RELIGIOUS TRAUMA

PDA (PATHOLOGICAL DEMAND AVOIDANCE)

MASKING

MELTDOWNS

SENSORY OVERWHELM

ARGUMENTS / DISAGREEMENTS

INCREASED TASKS

LACK OF SLEEP

STRESS

HORMONAL ISSUES

PERFECTIONISM

OVERUSING SPOONS

PARENTING DEMANDS

COMPLICATIONS FROM DISABILITIES / COMORBIDITIES

SUBSTANCE MISUSE

INCREASED PROBLEM BEHAVIORS

RSD (REJECTION SENSITIVE DYSPHORIA)

_____

_____

_____

@theautist

AUTISTIC SHUTDOWN PROFILE

COPING WITH MELTDOWNS
(CIRCLE YOURS)

● ● ● ● ● ●

SHOCK GROUNDING (LEMON, ORANGE, SALT, ETC.)
OTHER GROUNDING
MINDFULNESS
DEEP BREATHING
DEEP PRESSURE / HUGS
CO-REGULATION
NAPS / REST
STIMMING (LIST)

_____

_____

_____

OTHER (LIST)

_____

_____

_____

_____

_____

@therautist

AUTISTIC SHUTDOWN PROFILE

PLAN FOR SHUTDOWN
(CIRCLE YOURS)

●   ●   ●   ●   ●   ●

COUNSELING / THERAPY
EMDR, NEUROFEEDBACK, PLAY THERAPY, EQUINE THERAPY

ASK FOR SUPPORT
DELEGATE TASKS WHEN LIMITED ON SPOONS
REQUEST ACCOMMODATIONS AT WORK / SCHOOL
INCREASE REST
MINDFULNESS ACTIVITIES
FIND CONTENTMENT
LET GO OF SOMETHING'S

EXERCISE
YOGA, WALKS, HIKING, BIKING, RUNNING, ETC.

SELF-CARE
MASSAGES, MUSIC, REFLEXOLOGY, FLOATATION THERAPY,
ACUPUNCTURE, CHIROPRACTIC

SENSORY REGULATION
WEIGHTED BLANKETS, STIMMING, SOOTHING MUSIC

_____

_____

@theautist

AUTISTIC SHUTDOWN PROFILE

PLAN FOR SHUTDOWN
(CIRCLE YOURS)

● ● ● ● ● ●

BIG GUNS

RETREATS
-WITH SELF
-WITH SMALL GROUP
-MONASTERY

HOSPITILIZATIONS

WEEKEND GETAWAYS

_____

_____

_____

@theautist

Resources

Connect with me on Social Media

- https://www.facebook.com/TherAutist
- https://www.tiktok.com/@therautist
- https://twitter.com/TherAutist
- @AlliedCollaborative Facebook and Instagram
- https://www.facebook.com/kitchenscounseling/

Finding a Therapist

- https://www.psychologytoday.com

Recommended Books (Most are Autistic Authors)

- The Neurodivergent Friendly Workbook of DBT Skills by Sonny Jane Wise @livedexperienceeducator Facebook and Instagram
- Unmasking Autism by Devon Price
- Different Not Less by Chloe Hayden
- The Explosive Child by Dr. Ross Greene (Not autistic, but great information for parents and therapists in working with children and teens with the PDA profile)

- What I Mean When I Say I'm Autistic: Unpuzzling a Life on the Autism Spectrum by Annie Kotowicz @Neurobeautiful Facebook and Instagram
- I Will Die On This Hill by Meghan Ashburn and Jules Edwards
- Unusual Medicine Essays on Autistic Identity and Drug Addiction by David Gray-Hammond
- Untypical: How the World Isn't Built for Autistic People and What We Should All Do About It by Pete Wharmby

Autistic Autism Educators and Therapists to Follow on Social Media (There are so many and unfortunately I cannot list them all)

- @NeuroWild Facebook and Instagram
- @SpectrumSloth Facebook @kittysloth Instagram
- @TheAustisticTeacher Facebook
- @21andsensory Instagram
- @neurodivergent_insights Facebook and Instagram
- @livedexperienceeducator Facebook and Instagram

PDA Activists/Professionals to Follow
1. Kristy Forbes
   - Instagram @_kristyforbes
   - https://www.kristyforbes.com.au/
   - https://www.facebook.com/inTunePathways

2. Riko's PDA page
   - https://dragonriko.wordpress.com/
   - https://www.facebook.com/RikosPDApage1

3. Educating PDA
   - Instagram @educatingpda
   - https://www.facebook.com/educatingpda

4. Casey Ehrlich, Ph.D
   - Instagram @atpeaceparents
   - bio.site/atpeaceparents
   - https://www.facebook.com/atpeaceparents

Organizations to Follow

- NeuroClastic, Inc., is a 501(c)(3) non-profit organization and publication supporting autistic people and their families. They are a collective of neurodivergent people cataloging the experience, insights, knowledge, talents, and creative pursuits of autistics. www.neuroclastic.com

- The Autistic Self Advocacy Network (ASAN) is a 501(c)(3) nonprofit organization run by and for autistic people. The Autistic Self Advocacy Network seeks to advance the principles of the disability rights movement with regard to autism. ASAN believes that the goal of autism advocacy should be a world in which autistic people enjoy equal access, rights, and opportunities. We work to empower autistic people across the world to take control of our own lives and the future of our common community and seek to organize the autistic community to ensure our voices are heard in the national conversation about us. Nothing About Us, Without Us! http://www.autisticadvocacy.org/

Religious Trauma

- https://www.roomtothrive.com/resources

Trauma Therapy Modalities

1. EMDR
   - https://www.emdr.com/what-is-emdr/
   - https://www.emdria.org
   - How EMDR works? Look at this animation (English) https://youtu.be/hKrfH43srg8
   - EMDR: the weirdest therapy I've ever had https://youtu.be/J7KVJ8D0AM8

2. Neurofeedback
   - Neurofeedback Therapy Explained https://youtu.be/jqEJ53dwgNY

Rejection Sensitive Dysphoria

- Checklist and Self-test
  https://www.additudemag.com/rejection-sensitive-dysphoria-adhd-symptom-test/

SPECIAL THANKS AND ACKNOWLEDGMENTS

I am a big meme enthusiast and use them to express myself and add a flavor of humor to texts, emails, and general social media posts. I admit I also sometimes do this to prevent certain tones from being taken out of context. One meme comes to mind that I often share during Thanksgiving that I would love to put in here, and it includes a picture of a certain celebrity with a very unapproachable look that I am often guilty of myself. The meme states, "I am thankful for myself, for being myself." Of course, I say this in jest, but for this once, I am actually thankful for my ability to share a lot of my vulnerabilities because parts of it weren't easy. So, this meme actually fits for once. This ability got me through a project that I had not even set out to accomplish at the beginning of this year.

It goes without saying, but I definitely want to acknowledge my family and thank them for all the support they have given me all these years. I know I can get obsessive over certain topics and things when they spring up, and while autism and neurodiversity might not be one of your focused interests, you allow me to have it and info-dump on you at will. I am thankful for the support from my husband, Steven, in every endeavor I have ever set out to do. You have been nothing but positive and never tried to deter me from any of my crazy wild hairs. Whether they are going for an MBA or writing a book, you simply state, "Go for it." I know for a fact I wouldn't be where I am in this life without your support.

To my daughter, Kieran, thank you for sharing the gift of your voice for this audible book, as well as your editing and general English aptitude with your less-than-inept mother. I wish I had half of your talent. I know you will do great things with your writing in the future, and I cannot wait to see what you accomplish. To my three sons, Gage, Ryker, and Heston, thank you for putting up with my general obsessiveness and moodiness over the years, even when that obsessiveness becomes a project of redecorating your rooms. Thank you for giving me creative freedom, trusting me during the process and not complaining. To my youngest, Ridlee, thank you so much for teaching me what it means to unmask and let me be me. It was you who opened the door to find out who I truly was inside and gave me the answer for something that I was missing my whole life. To Carson, thank you for being a great son-in-law and loving my daughter as a husband should. And thank you for helping her with her editing duties. You and your mother, Kim, are both very dear to me, and I am so glad you both are in my life.

To my parents, thank you for everything. Thank you for showing me what a great example of what a good work ethic is. I know I wasn't the easiest child, but I am thankful for the parents that you were and for the love and support you always gave me. To my mom and my sister, Kelsey, thank you for validating many of my internal experiences on my journey toward my diagnosis. Sorry, I wasn't always the best big sister Kelsey. I know you still like to bring up the butter knife incident, and while I don't remember it, I don't doubt it happened at all. This is where I would insert a 'side eye monkey puppet" meme.

To two of my best friends and coworkers over the years, Ryan and Mark, thank you both for everything. Ryan, the last 18+ years have been incredible having you as a friend, raising our daughters close in age, playing roller derby together, going to grad school together, interning under you, and owning parallel practices. Our journeys have always lined up, and not once have we ever had a disagreement. You have supported me in every way and been my confidant without judgment through it all. Your advice is always sound, and your friendship means so much to me. I especially appreciate how I can go without contact for a bit and then pick up like no time ever passed. You are a true example of genuine friendship. Mark, thank you for always getting me and appreciating my special interest in Stevie Nicks. You come up with the most clever gifts that highlight my love for her. Thank you for trusting me over the years with work stuff and giving me wise counsel when needed. I have always valued your wisdom and positivity in everything. You are a great friend, and your family has been such a blessing to us.

Last but definitely not least, I do want to acknowledge my Lord and Savior, Jesus Christ. I know many have given you a bad rap. But I know the real Jesus and your love has brought me out of the darkest of holes, even when there was no hope in sight. Philippians 4:13, "I can do all things through Christ, who gives me strength," was my senior quote and has remained close to my heart during times of extreme sadness, pain, loss, and what I thought to be failures. But you made those failures into something better each and every time. I hope, despite my shortages and imperfections, that others can see your love through me. Thank you for laying this project on my heart and helping me bring it to fruition. Proverbs 16:3 says, "Commit your works to the Lord, and your plans will be established." I am committing this work to you, Lord, and I ask that you establish it to your will.

"For I will satisfy the weary soul, and every languishing soul will replenish." Jeremiah 31:25

About the Author

Jessica Kitchens,
MS, MBA, LPC, LADAC, MAC, RPT, BCCS

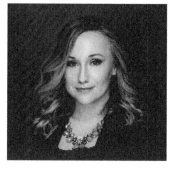

Jessica is an autistic private practice therapist in NW Arkansas. She has been married to her high school sweetheart for 24 years, and together, they have five children, one son-in-law, one grandchild, and three dogs. She has called NW Arkansas home for the past 20 years and has been a therapist for the past 15 of those. She specializes in working with autistic and other neurodivergent populations, as well as substance misuse, addictions, and play therapy. Outside of her own private practice, she also owns the first and only autistic-owned Neurodivergent-Affirming group counseling and consulting practice in NW Arkansas.

She holds a BA in Human Services Counseling, a dual MS in Marriage and Family Therapy and Community Counseling, and an MBA with an emphasis in Entrepreneurship. She is currently working towards a Ph.D. in Change Leadership for Equity and Inclusion, with an emphasis on Community Leadership and Change. Her indigenous heritage is very important to her as she is a tribal member of the Citizen Band Potawatomi nation.

In her spare time, she likes to research, read, write, run, hike, work out, dabble in arts and crafts on occasion, and spend time with her friends and family. Jessica has a strong love for working with neurodivergent individuals and hopes to make a brighter future for those in her community.

References

Arel, S. N. (2018). Disgust, shame, and trauma: The visceral and visual impact of touch. *Trauma and Lived Religion*, 45–70. https://doi.org/10.1007/978-3-319-91872-3_3

Arnsten, A. F. (2009). Stress signaling pathways that impair prefrontal cortex structure and function. *Nature Reviews Neuroscience, 10*(6), 410–422. https://doi.org/10.1038/nrn2648

Arnsten, A., Mazure, C. M., & Sinha, R. (2012). This is your brain in Meltdown. *Scientific American, 306*(4), 48–53. https://doi.org/10.1038/scientificamerican0412-48

ASAN. (2023). *Make real change on gun violence: Stop scapegoating people with mental health disabilities.* Autistic Self Advocacy Network. https://autisticadvocacy.org/policy/briefs/gunviolence/

Autistic people care too much, research says. NeuroClastic. (2020, July 11). Retrieved from https://neuroclastic.com/autistic-people-care-too-much-research-says/

Baron-Cohen, S. (1995). *Mindblindness: An essay on autism and theory of mind.* Boston: MIT Press/Bradford Books.

Belcher, H. (2022, July 7). *Autistic people and masking.* National Autistic Society. https://www.autism.org.uk/advice-and-guidance/professional-practice/autistic-masking

Brewer, N., Young, R. L., & Barnett, E. (2017). Measuring theory of mind in adults with autism spectrum disorder. *Journal of Autism and Developmental Disorders, 47*(7), 1927–1941. https://doi.org/10.1007/s10803-017-3080-x

Brown, A., Tse, T., & Fortune, T. (2018). Defining sensory modulation: A review of the concept and a contemporary definition for application by occupational therapists. *Scandinavian Journal of Occupational Therapy, 26*(7), 515–523. https://doi.org/10.1080/11038128.2018.1509370

Bruning, A. (2018, March 8). *Autistic panic attacks and meltdowns. which is which?* LinkedIn. https://www.linkedin.com/pulse/autistic-panic-attacks-meltdowns-which-allison-bruning

Cage, E., & Troxell-Whitman, Z. (2019). Understanding the reasons, contexts, and costs of camouflaging for autistic adults. *Journal of Autism and Developmental Disorders, 49*(5), 1899–1911. https://doi.org/10.1007/s10803-018-03878-x

Casanova, E. L., Baeza-Velasco, C., Buchanan, C. B., & Casanova, M. F. (2020). The relationship between autism and Ehlers-Danlos Syndromes/hypermobility spectrum disorders. *Journal of Personalized Medicine*, *10*(4), 260. https://doi.org/10.3390/jpm10040260

Champagne, T. (2008). *Sensory Modulation & Environment: Essential Elements of Occupation* (3rd Ed.). Southampton, MA: Champagne Conferences & Consultation.

Chapple, M., Davis, P., Billington, J., Myrick, J. A., Ruddock, C., & Corcoran, R. (2021). Overcoming the double empathy problem within pairs of autistic and non-autistic adults through the contemplation of serious literature. *Frontiers in Psychology*, *12*. https://doi.org/10.3389/fpsyg.2021.708375

Czech, H. (2018). Hans Asperger, National Socialism, and "Race Hygiene" in Nazi-era Vienna. *Molecular Autism*, *9*(1). https://doi.org/10.1186/s13229-018-0208-6

Cunha, J. P. (2022, August 23). *Neurotherapy: Definition, uses, benefits, and disadvantages.* eMedicineHealth. Retrieved January 26, 2023, from https://www.emedicinehealth.com/what_is_neurotherapy_for/article_em.htm

Datta, S. (2017, April 19). *Correcting hormonal imbalance may lead to improved quality of life for autistic individuals " autism 360™.* Autism 360™. https://www.autism360.com/news/correcting-hormonal-imbalance-may-lead-to-improved-quality-of-life-for-autistic-individuals/

Depression - autism: Autistica. Autistica. (2020, July 14). https://www.autistica.org.uk/what-is-autism/signs-and-symptoms/depression-and-autism

Dodson, W. (2022, July 11). *New insights into rejection sensitive dysphoria.* ADDitude. https://www.additudemag.com/rejection-sensitive-dysphoria-adhd-emotional-dysregulation/

Downie, A. (2022). Christian Shame and Religious Trauma. *Religions, 13*(10), 925. https://doi.org/10.3390/rel13100925

Emma, B. (2020, October 5). *Sensory trauma.* Undercover Autism. https://undercoverautism.org/2020/09/28/sensory-trauma

Fernández de la Cruz, L., Rydell, M., Runeson, B., Brander, G., Rück, C., D'Onofrio, B. M., Larsson, H., Lichtenstein, P., & Mataix-Cols, D. (2017). Suicide in Tourette's and chronic tic disorders. *Biological Psychiatry, 82*(2), 111–118. https://doi.org/10.1016/j.biopsych.2016.08.023

Forbes, K. (2020, April 27). *Intune Pathways - Kristy Forbes.* Kristy Forbes - Autism & Neurodiversity Support Specialist. https://www.kristyforbes.com.au/

Fox, A. (2019, January 22). *Post author: Reddoor.* Echolalia: The facts beyond "parrot talk", scripting, and echoing. https://reddoorpediatric.com/blog/echolalia-the-facts-beyond-parrot-talk-scripting-and-echoing/

Grant, R. (2023). *Robert Jason Grant, Ed.D: Mental Health and Education Services.* Robert Jason Grant Ed.D AutPlay® Therapy Clinic. https://www.robertjasongrant.com/

Gray-Hammond, D. (2022). Unusual Medicine Essays on Autistic Identity and Drug Abuse. David Gray-Hammond.

Groenman, A. (2022, April 27). *Menstruation and menopause in autistic people.* undefined. https://www.autism.org.uk/advice-and-guidance/professional-practice/menopause-menstruation

Groenman, A. P., Torenvliet, C., Radhoe, T. A., Agelink van Rentergem, J. A., & Geurts, H. M. (2021). Menstruation and menopause in autistic adults: Periods of importance? *Autism, 26*(6), 1563–1572. https://doi.org/10.1177/13623613211059721

Hayashi, M., Watanabe, M., & Hori, T. (1999). The effects of a 20 min nap in the mid-afternoon on mood, performance and EEG Activity. *Clinical Neurophysiology, 110*(2), 272–279. https://doi.org/10.1016/s1388-2457(98)00003-0

Higuera, V. (2021, November 19). *Rejection sensitive dysphoria: Causes, symptoms, and more.* Healthline. https://www.healthline.com/health/mental-health/rejection-sensitive-dysphoria

History and development: Brainworks Neurofeedback. Brainworks Neurofeedback | The UK's Neurofeedback leaders since 2007. London clinic, home training and industry software developers. (2022, November 12). https://brainworksneurotherapy.com/about/faq/history-and-development/

Hu, Y., Pereira, A. M., Gao, X., Campos, B. M., Derrington, E., Corgnet, B., Zhou, X., Cendes, F., & Dreher, J.-C. (2020). Right temporoparietal junction underlies avoidance of moral transgression in autism spectrum disorder. *The Journal of Neuroscience, 41*(8), 1699–1715. https://doi.org/10.1523/jneurosci.1237-20.2020

Hughes, C., Russell, J., & Robbins, T. W. (1994). Evidence for executive dysfunction in autism. *Neuropsychologia, 32*(4), 477–492. https://doi.org/10.1016/0028-3932(94)90092-2

Hull, L., Lai, M.-C., Baron-Cohen, S., Allison, C., Smith, P., Petrides, K. V., & Mandy, W. (2019). Gender differences in self-reported camouflaging in autistic and non-autistic adults. *Autism, 24*(2), 352–363. https://doi.org/10.1177/1362361319864804

Hum for your health: Why humming is so healing & how to do it. Flowly. (2022). https://www.flowly.world/post/hum-for-your-health-why-humming-is-so-healing-how-to-do-it

Jenkinson, R., Milne, E., & Thompson, A. (2020). The relationship between intolerance of uncertainty and anxiety in autism: A systematic literature review and meta-analysis. *Autism, 24*(8), 1933–1944. https://doi.org/10.1177/1362361320932437

Kelly, J. (2022, December 7). *The rise of the stay-at-home dad.* Forbes. https://www.forbes.com/sites/jackkelly/2022/12/07/the-rise-of-the-stay-at-home-dad

Khan, T. (2017, March 21). *Epilepsy and autism: Is there a relationship?* Epilepsy Foundation. https://www.epilepsy.com/stories/epilepsy-and-autism-there-relationship

Kinnaird, E., Stewart, C., & Tchanturia, K. (2019). Investigating alexithymia in autism: A systematic review and meta-analysis. *European Psychiatry, 55,* 80–89. https://doi.org/10.1016/j.eurpsy.2018.09.004

Kjellgren, A., & Westman, J. (2014). Beneficial effects of treatment with sensory isolation in flotation-tank as a preventive health-care intervention – a randomized controlled pilot trial. *BMC Complementary and Alternative Medicine, 14*(1). https://doi.org/10.1186/1472-6882-14-417

Kluger, J. (2023, January 6). *Perfectionists are at especially high risk for Burnout.* Time. https://time.com/6244829/burnout-mental-health-perfectionism/

Kupferstein, H. (2018). Evidence of increased PTSD symptoms in autistics exposed to applied behavior analysis. *Advances in Autism, 4*(1), 19–29. https://doi.org/10.1108/aia-08-2017-0016

LaiLin Yoga. (2019, June 4). *Practice point: Legs-on-a-chair pose.* LaiLin Yoga. https://www.lailinyoga.com.au/blog/2019/6/4/practice-point-legs-on-a-chair-pose

Mateos-Aparicio, P., & Rodríguez-Moreno, A. (2019). The impact of studying brain plasticity. *Frontiers in Cellular Neuroscience, 13*. https://doi.org/10.3389/fncel.2019.00066

Matusiak, M. (2020, January 29). *Autism and comorbid conditions*. Living Autism. https://livingautism.com/autism-comorbid-conditions/

McCrossin, R. (2022). Finding the true number of females with autistic spectrum disorder by estimating the biases in initial recognition and clinical diagnosis. *Children, 9*(2), 272. https://doi.org/10.3390/children9020272

Meier, S. M., Petersen, L., Schendel, D. E., Mattheisen, M., Mortensen, P. B., & Mors, O. (2015). Obsessive-compulsive disorder and autism spectrum disorders: Longitudinal and offspring risk. PLOS ONE, 10(11). https://doi.org/10.1371/journal.pone.0141703

Miller, J. (2022, October 31). *Autism and addiction*. Addiction Help. https://www.addictionhelp.com/addiction/autism/

Milton, D. (2020) *Neurodiversity Past and Present - an introduction to the Neurodiversity Reader.* In: Milton, Damian and Murray, Dinah and Ridout, Susy and Martin, Nicola and Mills, Richard, eds. The Neurodiversity Reader. Pavilion, Hove, UK, pp. 3-6. ISBN 978-1-912755-39-4.

Mitchell, P., Sheppard, E., & Cassidy, S. (2021). *Autism and the double empathy problem: Implications for development and ...*

Wiley Online Library. https://bpspsychub.onlinelibrary.wiley.com/doi/pdf/10.1111/bjdp.12350

Moreno, S. J. & O'Neal, C. (2000). Tips for teaching high functioning people with autism. Crown Point, IN: MAAP Services, Inc.

Myndlift. (2022, September 2). *A brief history of neurofeedback.* Myndlift. Retrieved from https://www.myndlift.com/post/2018/01/23/a-brief-history-of-neurofeedback

Newhouse, L. (2021, March 1). *Is crying good for you?* Harvard Health. https://www.health.harvard.edu/blog/is-crying-good-for-you-2021030122020

Newson, E., Maréchal, K., & David, C. (2003). Pathological demand avoidance syndrome: A necessary distinction within the pervasive developmental disorders. *Archives of Disease in Childhood, 88*(7), 595–600. https://doi.org/10.1136/adc.88.7.595

Nover, A. (2022, July 18). *Polycystic ovary syndrome associated with autism in mothers and children.* Psychiatry Advisor. https://www.psychiatryadvisor.com/home/topics/autism-spectrum-disorders/polycystic-ovary-syndrome-associated-with-autism-in-mothers-and-children/

Obaydi, H., & Puri, B. K. (2008). Prevalence of premenstrual syndrome in autism: A prospective observer-rated study. *Journal of International Medical Research, 36*(2), 268–272. https://doi.org/10.1177/147323000803600208

O'Connor, B. (2021, January 11). What causes double breathing after crying? Healthfully. https://healthfully.com/causes-double-breathing-after-crying-8384693.html

PDA - a guide for autistic adults. National Autistic Society. (2020). https://www.autism.org.uk/advice-and-guidance/topics/diagnosis/pda/autistic-adults

Pedersen, T. (2022, November 21). *Emotional dysregulation: Definition, signs, conditions, and coping.* Psych Central. https://psychcentral.com/blog/what-is-affect-or-emotion-dysregulation#definition

Pohl, A. L., Crockford, S. K., Blakemore, M., Allison, C., & Baron-Cohen, S. (2020). A comparative study of autistic and non-autistic women's experience of motherhood. *Molecular Autism, 11*(1). https://doi.org/10.1186/s13229-019-0304-2

Price, D. (2022). Unmasking Autism: Discovering the New Faces of Neurodiversity. Harmony Books.

Riko's blog: PDA and more. (2015). https://dragonriko.wordpress.com/

Robertson, J., Hatton, C., Emerson, E., & Baines, S. (2015). Mortality in people with intellectual disabilities and epilepsy: A systematic review. *Seizure, 29*, 123–133. https://doi.org/10.1016/j.seizure.2015.04.004

Rumball, F. (2022, March 30). *Post-traumatic stress disorder in autistic people.* National Autistic Society. https://www.autism.org.uk/advice-and-guidance/professional-practice/ptsd-autism

Rumball, F., Happé, F., & Grey, N. (2020). Experience of Trauma and PTSD Symptoms in Autistic Adults: Risk of PTSD Development Following DSM -5 and NON-DSM -5 Traumatic Life Events. Autism Research, 13(12), 2122–2132. https://doi.org/10.1002/aur.2306

Schultz, K. (2019, April 19). *What is spoon theory?* Healthline. https://www.healthline.com/health/spoon-theory-chronic-illness-explained-like-never-before#1

Simantov, T., Pohl, A., Tsompanidis, A., Weir, E., Lombardo, M. V., Ruigrok, A., Smith, P., Allison, C., Baron-Cohen, S., & Uzefovsky, F. (2021). Medical symptoms and conditions in autistic women. *Autism, 26*(2), 373–388. https://doi.org/10.1177/13623613211022091

Stanborough, R. J. (2021, November 19). *Understanding autism masking and its consequences.* Healthline. https://www.healthline.com/health/autism/autism-masking

Szalavitz, M., & Spectrum. (2017, March 2). *The hidden link between autism and addiction.* The Atlantic. https://www.theatlantic.com/health/archive/2017/03/autism-and-addiction/518289/

Theories about Autistic Experience. Aucademy. (2022, August 24). Retrieved April 5, 2023, from https://aucademy.co.uk/theories-about-autistic-experience/

Understanding the stress response. Harvard Health. (2020, July 6). https://www.health.harvard.edu/staying-healthy/understanding-the-stress-response

Verret, G. (2016, April 13). *Bullying and autism spectrum disorder (ASD): How to help your child.* Children's Hospital Los Angeles. https://www.chla.org/blog/rn-remedies/bullying-and-autism-spectrum-disorder-asd-how-help-your-child

Weintraub, K. (2019, March 25). *The adult brain does grow new neurons after all, study says.* Scientific American. Retrieved from https://www.scientificamerican.com/article/the-adult-brain-does-grow-new-neurons-after-all-study-says/

Weir, E., Allison, C., & Baron☒Cohen, S. (2021). The Sexual Health, orientation, and activity of autistic adolescents and adults. *Autism Research, 14*(11), 2342–2354. https://doi.org/10.1002/aur.2604

What is demand avoidance? PDA Society. (2022, October 29). https://www.pdasociety.org.uk/what-is-pda-menu/what-is-demand-avoidance/

What is eds? The Ehlers Danlos Society. (2023, January 23). https://www.ehlers-danlos.com/what-is-eds/

What is EMDR? (2020) EMDR. https://www.emdr.com/what-is-emdr/

Wilding, T. (2022, November 14). *What is demand avoidance, and when is it pathological?* Tomlin Wilding. https://

tomlinwilding.com/what-is-demand-avoidance-and-when-is-it-pathological/

YouTube. (2019, May 24). *Shrek Forever After (2010) - do the roar scene (3/10) | movieclips.* YouTube. https://www.youtube.com/watch?v=6I5B0jyLBUg&ab_channel=Movieclips

Printed in Great Britain
by Amazon

40513370R00126